The processes of aging and the challenges of life-thr   D0337649
cancer and heart disease are viewed through t
spirituality, poetry, mythology, and most of all, warm, grounded humanity.
Reading these essays I, a person navigating the mid-life passage while
facing down a particularly nasty type of cancer, felt less alone and more
connected to the legions of fellow travelers. I was inspired by stories of
courageous cancer survival, delighted by charming and utterly pragmatic
"tips" on how to successfully choose the "right" retirement home (start
looking years in advance, know your priorities, and have fun checking out
the possibilities), sobered by the reminder of the powerful role
psychological stress plays in heart health, and surprised and enlightened
by the idea of creating an ethical will (a document capturing one's values,
life lessons, wisdom, hopes and encouragements to share with our loved
ones). Above all, I felt empowered by the reminders that while so much of
what lies ahead is a mystery and beyond our knowing or control, there is
much that remains within our domain through the choices we make and
the stances we take. Anyone uncertain that beauty, grace, and wisdom can
be evoked from us through the aging process should read this book!

Thomas A. Potterfield, PhD
President, Institute of Transpersonal Psychology

As I grow older I find that two seemingly contradictory things are
happening. First, I am able to view things with much more objectivity than
when I was younger, and, second, I am able to enjoy and laugh at some
things I would have once found disturbing, even frightening. The authors in
this volume seem to have discovered much the same things, and it is a joy
to know that they are willing to share these with readers. Growing older is
so much easier when we can share both its joys and its challenges.

Wendy Nelder
Former President, San Francisco Board of Supervisors

This is an invaluable collection and synthesis of varied experiences,
perspectives, insights, and realistic approaches concerning the aging
process. Rarely do you find a riveting anthology; this one is, revealing a
wide variety of authentic experiences—all of which inspire hope, a sense of
earned freedom, and access to embodied wisdom, love, faith, and
acceptance found only in our later years. A "must read" for anyone over
fifty and for those who are care-givers at any age.

Angeles Arrien, PhD, Cultural Anthropologist, Sausalito, CA.
Author of *The Second Half of Life: Opening the Eight Gates of Wisdom*

Awakening to Aging is a deeply moving book. The contributors share with us their most profound experiences of aging and they write with both honesty and humor about coping with their own aging and with the aging and loss of beloved partners. The book will move you to laughter and to tears. It will remind you of the richness and the tremendous challenges that come late in life. Although aging and chronic illness might seem to focus on death, the contributors really celebrate life, love, and the everyday simple joys we too often forget.

Robert Frager, PhD
Founding President, Institute of Transpersonal Psychology, Palo Alto, CA

Residents in long-term elder care facilities often come to feel that they are in passive, receiving-only roles, a feeling which often leads to depression or anxiety which can then spread to other residents, caregivers and family members. This book is an antidote for such feelings, helping the elderly to focus on what they have to offer, to revitalize their gifts and discover new ones, and to once again experience that lift in self-esteem that comes from seeing oneself as a giver. As a therapist, I have benefited both personally and professionally from this book, which reminds all of us who are aware of our aging to stay in touch with the gifts aging brings.

John T. Bopp, PC, PhD
President, DBA Behavioral Health Systems
Kansas City, Missouri

Awakening to Aging addresses the aging process from a variety of perspectives. The introduction reminds us that as we live we get closer to death, becoming more acquainted with it as our contemporaries die from the various diseases of aging. As a physician, I can honestly say that we do not know much about health, for we tend to equate health with the absence of disease. Surely health is much more than that, as Barbara Sapienza expresses in her chapter, Cancer Koan. At 62 years of age I can now appreciate life from a very different perspective, and my life experience guides me in myriad ways. If we continue to celebrate life and the quality of life, then quantity may become less important, and it may be easier to "let go" when health declines beyond repair.

David Lakes, MD
Medical Oncologist, Kaiser Permanente, San Rafael, California,
Board Certified Hospice/Palliative Care specialist,
Assistant Clinical Professor, University of California, San Francisco

In *Awakening to Aging* editors Dr. Heery and Dr. Richardson have gathered a wide collection of authors bringing depth of knowledge and experience to the aging process. In his chapter, "Aging and Neurocognition," Richardson goes beyond scientific premise and with personal experience demonstrates examples of acceptance of the slow and not-so-slow inevitable. In the final chapter, "If You Live Long Enough," Heery gives a touching and insightful account of issues involved in aging and of the uncertainties in life and death, written with glimpses of the unknown which we all must face.

Albert M. Wall, MD, Savannah, Georgia

Most of us live our lives as if denial of aging and death is what keeps us going. Yet, the wisdom traditions counsel keeping the awareness of impermanence and change close at hand. The eighteen essays in *Awakening to Aging* do just this, inviting a glimpse of the inevitable with unparalleled skill, humor, and grace.

David Van Nuys, PhD
Emeritus Professor of Psychology, Sonoma State University
Producer of Shrink Rap Radio and Wise Counsel Podcasts

Themes of impermanence and awakening to the realities of both dying and living are gently woven through *Awakening to Aging.* Each chapter nudges us in the direction of awareness. This book offers multiple pathways and possibilities to navigate the still unknown. I left this book open to joy and to not-knowing, with the hope that I would be lucky enough to become old. With the quiet confidence of preparation, these stories can help us move gracefully into aging, death and dying. With the awareness and perspective of impermanence, we can move with the dignity and promise of truly living what they speak.

Gina Touch Mercer, PhD,
Assistant Professor, Clinical Psychology,
American School of Professional Psychology, Argosy University, Phoenix

These wise, informative and often poignant writings are treasures, reminders that the journey of our later years may be filled with anxiety, fear and decline, but also hold the possibility of being precious, enriching and surprising. One is inspired by these teachings to awaken to this final phase of life in wonderment and to live to the fullest, with gratitude and joy.

Margaret Hallett,
Executive Director, Family Service Agency of Marin, San Rafael, California

The authors not only share many professional and personal insights that help us better understand how and why we react to the loss of loved ones the way we do, but just as important, especially for the lay reader, provide many helpful tools for coping with those losses.

Jeff Richardson
Former Secretary, Indiana Family Social Services Administration

A timely book—Myrtle Heery and Gregg Richardson have gathered authors from diverse backgrounds to provide a broad range of topics that inform, awaken, and provide wisdom for our journey through this last stage of life.

Ann Coffey, PhD
Director and CO-founder with Elizabeth Bugental, PhD of Agesong,
a program for seniors at Family Service Agency of Marin, San Rafael, CA

Written primarily for Baby Boomers, *Awakening to Aging: Glimpsing the Gifts of Aging* covers a broad spectrum of aging issues as it attempts to move and guide those of us in this vast post-WWII generation. Editors Myrtle Heery PhD and Gregg Richardson PhD have gathered an esteemed group of writers who share not only their professional gerontological expertise, but more importantly, their heartfelt and personal insights into their own aging processes. "Awakening to Aging" comes at the right time. Baby boomers are simultaneously retiring and caring for parents, spouses, siblings, and friends. Amidst these stressful role changes, we are also facing an uncertain future with our health care system. Many of us wonder if we will have the financial and psychological resources to age well. This book offers practical advice as well as much hope. It soothes us with its affirmation of the transcendent wisdom that can be found in later life, while it compels us to face our own aging with pride and honesty.

Moira Keller, LCSW
Geriatric Care Manager, Sixty Plus Older Adult Services
Piedmont Hospital, Piedmont, GA

As a hospital staff nurse who cares for an increasingly aged population, I was encouraged to read about many of the problems our patients have to tackle. I often wonder how they were managing at home before they came through our doors on a gurney or in a wheelchair. These chapters cover the multifaceted challenges of aging in a clear and logical format. It is a genuine resource for caregivers of all health care disciplines.

Gina Leoni, RN, BSN
Medical Surgical Nurse, Palm Drive Hospital, Sebastopol, CA

In my work as a hospice nurse it is rare that I encounter a person that is prepared for the process of dying. This book explores this problem with the gentleness that is necessary in order to approach such a grand and intimidating journey—the end of life.

Deborah Quevedo, RN, PhD, San Jose, CA

Awakening to Aging:
Glimpsing the Gifts of Aging

Edited by
Myrtle Heery &
Gregg Richardson

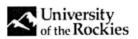 **University**
of the **Rockies**

University of the Rockies Press
555 E. Pikes Peak Avenue, #108
Colorado Springs, Colorado 80922

This book is dedicated in memory of the editors'
beloved parents and teachers.

B.B. and Camille Heery
&
Tom and Marian Richardson

Jim and Elizabeth Bugental
&
Hobart "Red" and Rachel Thomas

Table of Contents

Part 4: GIFTS OF WISDOM - AWAKENING TO THE UNKNOWN

Acknowledgments

My deepest gratitude to each and all of the transparent authors in this book—Elizabeth Bugental, Carol Cook, Doug Cort, Pamela Cronin, Karuna Gerstein, Christopher Grimes, Sandra Harner, Fran Korb, John Levy, Laura Michaels, Bev Miller, Regina Reilly, Will Rogers, Barbara Sapienza, and Hobart "Red" Thomas. Their words are the gifts of aging for you, the reader.

And to my co-editor and author, Gregg Richardson, who inspired me as he moved his parents from Ohio to his home in Berkeley, California, during the last decade of their lives. Both died during the process of our producing this book. Thank you Gregg for standing by your parents and this book from start to finish with clarity of mind and open heart.

It is easy to let manuscripts sit and get dusty as we get consumed with other tasks. This one certainly did. But then I showed a video clip of one of our Awakening to Aging seminars at a professional training, Unearthing the Moment. My dear friend and colleague, Louis Hoffman, was there and was very moved, but unlike most people who are moved by video clips, Louis is one of those who acts on such feelings. You would not be reading this book if Louis and the University of the Rockies Press had not come forward to publish this manuscript. Thank you.

In addition to Louis's wonderful editing skills, we were blessed to have the talents of his staff, including Angela Nazworth, who refined these chapters with her sensitive editing, and Laura Ross, who worked with my photograph to make a memorable cover for all to appreciate.

Marla Zahira Rabinowitz produced our wonderful bibliography and supported our progress by asking regularly, "How is it going?" Richard Applegate edited as needed and his benevolent advice was always heeded.

A loving thank you to my dear Aunt Lucille and my close friend Connie Mahoney (both turned 90 in 2009) for unremitting wisdom generously given to me.

Over a dozen reviewers from across the United States generously gave of their time and support for this book, and their moving words are deeply appreciated.

I must also thank my husband, William, who beat the odds with metastatic melanoma and lived to raise our son, Jamie, with me. Jamie graduated from college and got a job during the making of this book. To both of you, who did not know half the time what I was doing and the other half supported me with questions, perceptions, computer skills, and great jokes, thank you both.

Two of our authors, Elizabeth Bugental and Hobart "Red" Thomas, as well as their spouses, Jim Bugental and Rachel Thomas, died before this book was published, but in its formative stages, each was instrumental in moving the book forward. Elizabeth introduced me to two people who went on to contribute to the book, John Levy and Karuna Gerstein. Red was always available for a what-to-do-next session. Jim told me often that the book would come out at just the right time, and those words of wisdom have proven true as debates over a new health care bill in the U.S. intensifies and this book goes to press. We dedicate this book to each of you and to our parents, B.B. and Camille Heery and Tom and Marian Richardson.

Finally, I want to thank mysterious nature, for birds splashing in birdbaths, roses blooming, waves crashing, and so many other daily reminders of both beauty and impermanence. Thank you.

To the board and advisory board of our International Institute for Humanistic Studies (IIHS), which sponsored and continues to sponsor educational dialogues on *Awakening to Aging,* thank you! Without these educational dialogues, this book would not exist. For ongoing information about Awakening to Aging please contact IIHS through www.human-studies.com, mheery@sonic.net, or 707-763-3808, ext. 2.

M.H.

Foreword

Gregg Richardson

A unique set of circumstances makes this volume of essays possible. First, assuming that the human population has been more or less steadily increasing, apart from some losses to the plague, since we first appeared on the planet, and that we are generally living longer than our predecessors (at least since the beginning of the scientific age), we can now legitimately claim to have more people over the age of 50 than ever before. This is especially true in the United States given that after World War II thousands of lonely soldiers returned to equally lonely spouses and produced the Baby Boom. It was predetermined that a large cohort of the United States population would now be reaching retirement age and facing the various medical, emotional, financial, and social problems encountered by older people in this country.

Second, technology now makes it possible for virtually anyone in the First World (and increasingly in the Third World), to communicate instantly by phone or e-mail. Facts, ideas, and images can be shared as soon as they appear. Amateur videos can alter the outcome of court cases. And even professional reporters and researchers rely on the Internet and private cell phones for instant information.

Third, advances in medicine and technology have made it possible, at least for most of us, to live longer and healthier lives than our parents (and certainly our ancestors, for whom 40 was an advanced age). The pains of arthritis are reduced, joints are replaced, hearts can be artificially paced, and cancers kept under control for years. And those diseases and debilitations that have not yet been made tolerable are increasingly the focus of research and invention as the market for their management grows.

The result of these and other factors is that there are many aging individuals in the United States and elsewhere who are able and motivated to share their experiences and insights about aging, to help one another on this journey that goes in only one direction (or stops), and to make it as pleasant and fulfilling as possible. The contributors to this volume all view aging from different perspectives and believe that sharing those perspectives is a key to improving the journey for all of us. We offer you our experiences and insights, the little wisdoms we have each garnered over the years, and invite you to use them in your own awakening to aging.

Introduction

I remember sitting at the feet of my grandmother watching her fingers move quickly, pulling fine threads through the needle, creating the most beautiful table mat I had ever seen. She was crocheting. I was five years old. We sat on the big screen porch of our summer home at Savannah Beach, Georgia, a home the locals called "Tybee." A typical humid 100-degree day would bring our afternoons to a languid halt. We would use fans to cool off and swat mosquitoes with tightly rolled papers. Boredom was part of those hot afternoons. Some would read, others sleep, but I would watch Grannie crochet.

I looked forward to those hot afternoons, when I would have Grannie all to myself in the still heat. I loved this little old lady with the innocence of a child chasing a butterfly. I was fascinated by her fingers and hands, so strong and quick. I remember being able to see the veins under her thin skin, veins I could not see under my own, which was all smooth. I couldn't understand this, but knew that Grannie would.

"Grannie, how come I can see the veins in your hands and not in mine?"

"Oh child, not to worry. When you age you too will see the veins in your hand."

In one quick sentence I awakened to aging! I would be aging when I could see the veins in my hands! How amazing! Well, I see the veins in my hands clearly now. I am sixty-three, still not Grannie's age when I asked her that question, but very much awake to aging, and my awakening continues.

Perhaps those veins showing themselves to me and the world are one of the first signals that life is not moving as smoothly as Grannie's hands moved the thread. Life is taking its toll, and life's thinness becoming much more tangible. As I run my fingers over my visible veins I feel the full range of loss of grandparents, parents, aunts, uncles, teachers, and many dear friends long gone, and recognizing that I too am aging and moving toward the end of my aging, my death.

I am a Baby Boomer, part of the largest population that has ever aged. Baby Boomers, if you are hoping to find out how to stop aging, this is *not* the book for you. If you are looking for facts and stories that wake you up to the emotional realities of aging, then this book *is* for you.

We use the term "awakening" in two ways in this book, first as an opening to a larger view of self and life brought about by simply waking up to the physical fact of aging, and second in the more Buddhist sense of awakening to one's true nature, of developing a transparent presence of being. Both are woven into the personal stories collected in this book.

The essence of aging is found in paradox, particularly for the Baby Boomers who seem so determined to beat the "d word," death, an effort that often turns to poignant surrender. As a dear childhood friend, Kirk Varnedoe, former curator of the MOMA in New York City, said at the end of his last slide presentation at the Smithsonian three months before his death at 54 from colon cancer: "There it is. I have shown it to you. It has been done. It is being done. And because it can be done, it will be done. And now I am done" (Varnedoe, 2006, p. 272).

Some of us will not be done for awhile. This gives us the gift of time—to prepare, to choose, to find meaning in the time we have left, to leave our mark, to explore more closely and with humility the mysteries of living and dying. But gifts imply both giving and receiving, and are associated not only with holidays or birthdays but also with emotions ranging from joy to disappointment. My mother had a special section in a closet where she kept "recycled gifts" to be used on future occasions. Unfortunately, she never marked who had given a particular gift. Inevitably, she once gave, to a dear friend on her birthday, the same gift she had received from this woman many years ago. Needless to say, the friend was insulted, but in time the tension between them transformed into an ongoing joke about how that returned gift was a part of their long and treasured friendship.

Aging can resemble this recycled gift closet, where unwanted gifts of aging are stored. The personal stories and facts in this book may become gifts you choose to store or share, but we hope they will stand by you like old friends as you awaken to aging, gently reminding you, as old friends do so well, to laugh.

The personal and the factual are interwoven both in our actual aging and in this book. We have organized them here into four major categories: gifts shared—leaving the known; gifts returned—the mind and body; gifts for the journey—walking the talk; and gifts of wisdom—awakening to the unknown. We offer both personal and professional accounts of gifts once received that we each must give back as we age—money, property, position, body, mind, emotions, caregiving—and when all seems finally to be gone and we lie naked in our prison of aging, we are then given the gift of wisdom, the multidimensional voice of spirit.

Seventeen different authors walk beside you and share their wisdom about aging. Some emphasize the facts of aging, others share their personal stories about aging. We need both as we now heatedly debate the future of health care in America. The emotional questions and the shouted answers at town hall meetings are not the summer of Woodstock but the summer of Healthstock! It is time to take stock of the realities of aging in this country. Will we pay for our bodily dysfunctions as we age, and how? These authentic authors address the underbelly of these issues—the high monetary, emotional and spiritual costs of aging.

This book invites emotional and spiritual answers that are not shouted but rather offered gently, thoughtfully, with a hand on your shoulder, as in the cover photograph of Dr. and Mrs. Chaun. The words in this book bring facts that resonate with the authenticity of experience and insight. These authors invite you to awaken to aging with hope, courage, and ultimately surrender to the last gift of aging, death.

Paradoxically, awakening to aging is a process of accepting impermanence and the ultimate surrender of the greatest gift, our life itself. This process of surrendering, of giving back all that we have known and leaning into the unknown dimensions of spirit can be heard in the voice of William Shakespeare's King Lear:

> "No, no, no, no! Come, Let's away to prison:
> We two alone will sing like birds i'the cage;
> When thou dost ask me blessing, I'll kneel down
> And ask of thee forgiveness: so we'll live,
> And pray, and sing, and tell old tales, and laugh
> At gilded butterflies, and hear poor rogues
> Talk of court news and we'll talk with them too, --
> Who loses and who wins; who's in, who's out; --
> And take upon's the mystery of things,
> As if we were God's spies: and we'll wear out,
> In a wall'd prison, packs and sects of great ones,
> That ebb and flow by th'moon."
> (Shakespeare, *King Lear*, Act IV, scene III, p.245)

Prayers, songs, laughter, the telling of tales, all ripened by age, a passing-on of the wisdom learned in simply being alive. The great gift of aging is to pass on wisdom to those yet to age.

These stories developed primarily from panels, starting in 2004, in which various helping professionals discussed aging with other professionals as part of continuing education and lay people of various ages and cultures. These panels were and are sponsored by the International Institute for Humanistic Studies (www.human-studies.com), a non-profit organization dedicated to building bridges of communication among cultures through compassion, courage, hope, resilience, and tolerance. We hope that these facts and stories become gifts of wisdom for you as you too awaken to aging.

Myrtle Heery
Petaluma, California
August, 2009

References

Shakespeare, W. (2005). *The tragedy of King Lear* (Jay L. Halio, Ed.), Cambridge, England: Cambridge University Press.

Varnedoe, K. (2006). *Pictures of nothing*. Princeton, N.J.: Princeton University Press.

Part 1

Gifts Shared:
Leaving the Known

1

Living the Facts:
The Largest Aging Population

Pamela Cronin

When I wrote my Master's Thesis in 1996 on *Life Satisfaction and the Aging Population*, I realized that at some point I would revisit the issues of aging from a personal, family, friend, and community perspective. Over the past decade, I have observed the aging process most directly in myself, my family, and my friends. In this chapter, I want to examine how the changes in my life are similar to those of millions of people throughout the world. This research, completed in the 1990s, is still relevant today.

Aging Facts

The "graying of America" refers to the fact that an ever-greater proportion of the U.S. population is comprised of senior citizens. This growth in the aging population has been attributed to various factors— increasing longevity, a declining birth rate among younger persons (Kinney & Leaton, 1991, as cited in the Mosby Year Book, 1991), advanced medical technology, and increased health awareness in the elderly leading to improved self-care (Statistics Bureau, Management, and Coordination Agency, 1988).

In 1900 there were approximately 123,000 persons in The United States who surpassed 85 years of age. Today there are more than three million. By 2050 some predict that there will be as many as 50 million, representing more than 16 percent of the population (Bortz, 1991). According to the U.S. Bureau of the Census (1991), the number of people older than age 65 increased from around 11 percent in 1980 to approximately 16 percent by the year 2000. Canada's senior population is expected to sharply increase from its current 12 percent to approximately 25 percent by the year 2026 (Hawranik & Walker, 1995).

Sweden, Germany, Japan, and the United States lead the list of developed countries faced with burgeoning elderly populations; and researchers indicate that the average age and lifespan of individuals in these nations will continue to increase. Japan's Ministry of Health and Welfare indicates that the average ages of 76.11 years for men and 82.11 years for women are at an all-time high due to increased medical technology and health awareness among the aging (Statistics Bureau, Management, and Coordination Agency, 1988).

In the United States, according to the Health Insurance Association of America (HIAA), life expectancy at birth is 71.5 for males and 78.3 for females (HIAA, 1991). Kenneth Manton (1982), a scholar and demographer of aging at Duke University, has calculated that 1% of all males and females born in America in 1975 will live for 105 years and 110 years, respectively (cited in Woodbury, et al., 1982).

Based on statistical information on aging in the U.S. provided by an Experience Corps fact sheet on aging in America (Civic Ventures, www.civicventures.org), some of the 1996 statistics mentioned are low by today's standards. They believe that in the year 2000 there were 34.8 million people (12% of the population) over the age of 65. Their projections for 2030 predict 70.3 million people over the age of 65 years, representing 20% of the population.

The likelihood that an American who reaches the age of 65 will survive to the age of 90 has nearly doubled over the past forty years. By 2050 it is estimated that 40% of 65-year-olds will likely live to age 90.

Message of the Facts

As more people live longer, the United States will not be alone in facing a formidable challenge in paying for the care of our elders.

This raises the question of how we are going to care for ourselves independently or with a spouse as we move toward retirement. It is therefore more important than ever to have a plan for our golden years. If we continue to rely on government assistance, we will find ourselves in line with millions of others competing for the same care, which may or may not be available due to skyrocketing health care costs.

Despite predictions that the next generation of retirees will be the healthiest, longest lived, best educated, and most affluent in history, current 65-year-olds reported a median income of $32,854 in 2000.

This income is lowest for Hispanics ($24,330), with African Americans in the middle ($27,952), and Caucasians at the top ($33,467).

The good news is that more retirees are healthier for longer and choose to remain in the work force longer. More retirees also volunteer and help other elders to navigate the system (2004, Experience Corps).

Social Considerations on Aging

Some contributing social factors with psychological impact were seen in Beattie's 1986 study (cited in Keith, 1986), which concluded that as the elderly population grows, we can expect an increase in the proportion of the unmarried population who need more health care and other services than married elders. This study looked at factors associated with isolation among widowed, divorced, separated, and never-married individuals, and found that men and women in these groups generally suffered more isolation from neighbors and friends than from family (although the never-married maintained more ties with friends). Divorced and never-married men were more isolated from family than were widowed men, while women's isolation from family differed less by marital status than that of men (Keith, 1986). According to Borges et al. (1984), women expected future levels of satisfaction to be higher than did men.

Another factor contributing to life satisfaction among elders is their dating relationships. One study suggested that most older persons place greater emphasis on companionship than on passion in relationships (Bulcroft & O'Connor, 1986). While older women felt that dating increased their prestige, older men stressed the importance of dating as a means for self-disclosure; the authors concluded that dating in later life is a hedge against loneliness.

Life Satisfaction and Aging

Erik H. Erikson's (1959) eight stages of psychosocial and psychosexual development is a theoretical approach to understanding the needs of the aging population and the balance required to integrate and stabilize the ego's role in the individual's life history.

Erikson believed that the healthy person is one who is able to work and love, i.e., one who has the capacity to share intimacy with another and to work fruitfully and with personal satisfaction. Given a healthy parental and social environment, the individual develops a sense of ego integrity. This involves the development of "all that the person is, unique capacities, and the complete acceptance of self, for better or worse" (Erikson, 1967, as cited in Monte, 1991, p.293).

In Erikson's view, the first seven stages influence the eighth and final stage, Integrity vs. Despair (Erikson, 1959). In his view, old age sees a return to the playfulness of childhood in the wise elder's affirmation of the life he or she has led (Monte, 1991).

The literature indicates that the elderly report different levels of satisfaction with their lives, and a number of variables affecting this satisfaction were found in the literature. Wolkenstein and Butler (1992) provided important data in a survey research project designed to describe the quality of life in seniors over the age of 65 years who maintained activities of daily living (ADLs) in their own apartments within a retirement community for socially functioning healthy elders. Two surveys and lectures on health and nutrition were used on a majority of elderly Caucasian women between the ages of 71 and 90 years. Quality of life was defined in three ways: a) the outer world, b) the inner self, and c) the ability to cope with loss. The surveys assessed their ability to perform physical activities, physical independence, self-esteem, satisfaction, attitude toward life, self-sufficiency, and the process of coping with loss at their stage of life. The results suggested, most importantly, that quality of life was important to the elderly group. Some perceived their coping skills to be the same as other age groups while others felt they had come to the end of the road with fewer resources and less time to adjust to the changes in their lives. Their responses suggested that they wanted physicians to become more involved with the whole person, not simply the ailing parts.

Much of the literature tends to have fewer male respondents. Researchers refer to the uneven distribution of respondents involving life satisfaction, and the most often possible cause cited is the fact that women tend to have greater longevity than men (Borges et al., 1984; Bulcroft & O'Connor, 1986; Caserta et al., 1993).

Borges et al. (1984) rated the current, past, and projected future life satisfaction of 432 people in six age groups. They found that the average ratings for men and women did not differ, although women tended to judge the age interval prior to their own, as well as their present age interval, as less satisfying than did men. However, women expected future levels of life satisfaction to be higher than did men. The researchers concluded that "this optimism is attributed to socialization differences as well as the hope engendered by the current feminist movement" (Borges et al., 1984).

Nutrition, Emotions, and Physical Activity

Nutrition is another important area of research to be considered when working with the aging population. Ahmed (1992), in an archival research project for the Food and Nutrition Board, analyzed 76 previous studies on the effects of malnutrition and lack of vitamins and minerals on the health of the elderly. He concluded that poor nutrition may play a significant role in the progressive decline of body functions with aging. The effects of nutrition on aging are significant because malnutrition affects the progress of many degenerative diseases such as osteoporosis, cardiovascular disease, and some forms of cancer. Approximately 75 percent of all deaths, and half of all bed-confinement days among the elderly are attributable to chronic degenerative diseases.

Malnutrition in older adults results from primary causes such as poverty, isolation, ignorance of the need for a balanced diet, and alcohol and other drug abuse. Ahmed (1992) theorizes that because aging is a lifelong process, diminished physical activity and old-age disabilities cause the elderly to modify eating habits acquired at a young age. Depression may then occur and a vicious cycle ensues. He concluded that to enjoy a better mental and physical quality of life, dietary and other lifestyle changes, such as exercise habits, should be established early in the life cycle so that optimal tissue and physical functioning will be maximally maintained into the latest years.

Chapuy et al. (1992) concurred with Ahmed's evaluation of the effects of calcium and vitamins on the elderly. They concluded that fractures can be substantially reduced with the simple addition of calcium and vitamin intake to the diet.

Good health and physical activity have been associated with successful aging. Roos and Havens (1991) reported in their 12-year longitudinal study that remaining independent (defined as being able to perform ADLs) was associated with a higher level of life satisfaction, although it did not guarantee life satisfaction in advanced age. Despite the limitations of several contradictory analyses of the multiple factors involved in the survey, the data clearly suggested that healthy and active older adults expressed a higher level of life satisfaction.

Loneliness has many forms for older people and can initiate health and emotional problems if ignored. Individuals who enjoyed independence and privacy in young adulthood may experience feelings of isolation in later years as needs and activities change. Retirement from the work force, loss of family and friends, and a decrease in social connections and activities are transitions that can lead to solitude and a vicious cycle of loneliness and despair. The greatest challenge in combating loneliness is having the older individual take the first step toward communicating with others; no one else can do this for him or her. A belief that each person has something to offer others and a willingness to take some emotional risks are central to reaching out and becoming involved with groups and organizations. Frequently these steps result in new friendships and stronger ties with the community (Lutz et al., 1990).

Lutz et al. (1990) with the University of California School of Medicine, San Francisco, developed a significant guidebook on the aging process for the California Department of Mental Health, Office of Prevention. The guide examines the realities of growing old and dispels some of the myths of aging. A common myth about sexuality and aging, for example, is that the physical changes of aging reduce sexual appetite and ability, and that sex is for the young. The reality is that our society does not often acknowledge the sexual needs of older adults, resulting in many seniors hiding their sexual desires. Sexual problems can occur at any age and conditions affecting sexuality may be treatable. The guide lays out the myths and realities of aging in a comprehensive and easy to read style. A section on 'lifestyle choices' discusses the benefits of good nutrition, regular exercise, enhancing social support, increasing enjoyable and meaningful activities, becoming assertive, and decreasing tension through deep relaxation.

The 'common challenges' facing seniors are illness and disability, financial insecurity, life transitions, reduced memory, care needs, the possibility of elder abuse, medication problems, falls, sexual needs, grieving, sight and hearing impairment, stress, depression, and embracing their mortality. Professional references are included for those seeking further information and education on the aging process. It is an excellent resource tool that provides positive and realistic assistance, solutions, and most importantly, hope, for the aging population (Lutz et al. 1990).

Living the Facts

In 2003, I discovered that my then 84-year-old mother was suffering from depression, but that as an apparently independent, strong Irish matriarch she was hiding her "shameful" mental condition from family and friends. In Ireland one still frequently finds the notion that it is far better to secretly battle the demons of the mind than to seek counseling. She was in fact seeing her physician on a regular basis and was covertly being treated with antidepressants, but her doctor, over the course of two years, based upon her reports of the "tablets not agreeing with her," frequently changed her medications. Unbeknownst to him, she would try the medications for a week or two, then stop taking them because "they didn't do her any good at all." She saved the unused medications, however, and if she felt "down" would often take the oldest of these, rationalizing that they were probably better than the newer, but in general took what fancied her as though sampling a box of assorted chocolates. This dangerous practice began to affect her mental well-being and finally her doctor, in frustration, referred her to a psychiatrist. He believed she was one of those unsolvable cases. My mother eventually suffered a severe major depressive episode and we as a family rushed to the rescue. I decided that I needed to gather some facts before meeting with my seven siblings.

I traveled to Dublin, Ireland, in the autumn of 2003 and spent several weeks listening to and talking with my mother, her psychiatrist, and her physician. After a thorough medical investigation and psychiatric assessment, we removed all medications from her home and all prescriptions were eventually stopped. She was admitted to a Seniors Group where on a weekly basis depressed seniors could share their insights and issues. After our initial visit to the center my mother indicated that she did not wish to join a group of old depressed people. It was an interesting observation on her part. She was unable to see her own level of depression.

My perspective was quite different when I realized that my mother would be one of the oldest participants and wondered if she would be accepted by the younger group members. I decided that my strong and capable mother of yesteryear did not recognize her aging process and was desperately fighting her fear of her own mortality. Many of her friends had either died or moved away, and feelings of isolation were beginning to have their effect. Grief and loss counseling, and openly processing one's own mortality, are still unknown in many parts of the "new" Ireland. I recalled childhood memories of funerals and wakes with my grandparents and parents, where death and dying were celebrated with parties and story-telling about the deceased. Music was played, songs sung between libations, and food eaten for the departed soul. Poetry and significant literary pieces were read, and jokes and laughter were as common as tears of loss and wails of sadness. The old country's culture celebrated death, embracing rather than fearing it. Ten years after completion of my MA thesis on *Life Satisfaction and the Aging Population* I was confronted with my mother's declining health, causing me to examine mortality more generally—my mother's, my family's, my friends', my own.

I discovered over the following weeks that my mother was ambivalent about how or where she wanted to live the remainder of her life. At times when we talked about her thoughts and feelings, she was clear that remaining alone in her small, comfortable two-storey home on a quiet cul-de-sac outside the city was not a long-term option. She could, however, envision her 90-year-old sister and herself living in a nice retirement community. Then within hours she would revert to not knowing what she wanted. I drove the sisters all over the county of Dublin looking at potential retirement communities. It was amazing to hear them process the pros and cons of each place. Mostly they criticized the facilities, the staff, and the residents. It was clear that we were not going to find that heavenly spot in Ireland. I found myself thinking about my clients and how difficult it is for the children of aging parents to cope with their inability to find closure.

As the oldest daughter and second of eight siblings, I began to realize that my skills as a therapist, working with other families dealing with elderly/parental problems, were not of value within my own family. My five brothers (all living in Europe) emerged the obvious leaders of the patriarchy, and each had unique solutions to mother's problems. I listened to strong words of denial of her aging process, her depression, her mortality, and her fears. Some solutions they offered were to sit her down and discuss the matter in a very rational way, to get her to see the reality of her situation, to not let her talk negatively about issues, to have her live with one or more of us throughout the year, to let her enjoy a nice glass of Irish whiskey, to let her make all her own decisions as she had always done, and so on. One brother was so incensed that I, the lone American, was the instigator of trouble when in fact our mother did not even need the safety bar for the bathtub and stairs recommended by a visiting social worker. It began to register with me that they, too, were unwilling to look at either our mother's mortality or their own.

My sisters and I along with several of my sisters-in-law were more realistic about the situation. We agreed that my mother, widowed at 39 years of age and who had raised us alone, had no desire to leave her own house. She loved her children and her own space and freedom, and we realized that we were all in a double-bind of my mother's creation. She listened to her sons' desire to believe there was nothing to worry about, but complained to the women about her loneliness and life challenges.

Five years later the situation remains status quo. Safety bars were installed in the home and family members visit as frequently as possible, albeit often from long distances. Telephone trees are established and she speaks to several family members each week. She attends her seniors group, enjoys chatting to the old folk, visits with her sister and her family, and continues to experience different levels of depression and a new level of forgetfulness. At times, she becomes frustrated with herself as she reaches for the appropriate words. She will not discuss the notion of a will/trust, her death, or where her burial site should be. Her children and family continue to live in a state of suspense, knowing that one day we will have to deal with her death. The reality of her situation has softened some of the denial around her frailty. There is more acknowledgment from my brothers that our mother is in need of more care and we try to assist her differently as we recognize her decline. We are more accepting that our mother wants to remain in her home until she decides what to do. We are respectful of her wishes and needs and know that in all likelihood she will stay at home until she dies.

My story is but one of millions of similar stories emerging as the elder population increases.

Younger generations are often faced with the dilemma of caring for an ailing or terminally ill parent. I have encountered individuals 40-plus years-old, on a fast career track, raising children and building a future for themselves and their families, who have to find the financial and health resources to accommodate the needs of their parents'. Some are willing and financially able to assist parents by having them live in their homes with them, while others want to place them in assisted-living or nursing homes. Parents find themselves in a situation they had not planned for, and settle for what is available—financially, emotionally, spiritually. There are many elders in nursing facilities who are unhappy and waiting to die.

Cultural differences play a huge part in family caretaking. A Filipino daughter was charged with caring for her mother in her own home with three small children. Her adult brothers were all dependent on their mother emotionally and financially and did not know how to cope with her long-term kidney dysfunction and eventual dialysis. Over time, the daughter and other members of the family taught the adult sons to participate and assist with their mother's care, and she lived comfortably with her daughter until her death four years later. Her sons learned to become financially and emotionally independent, and today the extended family is closer because of their experience and their need to adjust to life's circumstances.

Other cases abound where families are torn apart because siblings differ on what should be done with a parent. They attempt various strategies. They try sharing care, for example, but over time resentments develop when one feels unfairly burdened.

Often the parent has no say in matters, no chance to express what he or she wants or feels. Parent and child roles switch and emotional and spiritual support is lost or becomes chaotic as each individual attempts to cope with the stress and anxiety overload. The question of mortality is frequently left unaddressed as the family watches a loved one die.

There is no doubt in my mind that as more people live longer, there will be a greater need for all types of services, including housing, senior care facilities, mental and physical health programs, support groups, medical care facilities, and most important, family care providers. I believe that as government health care becomes less available and more costly due to escalating numbers of elders, families will be faced with absorbing and solving more of the elder care issues. It will be interesting to observe the inevitable changes we face over the next decades—socially, medically, and politically.

References

Adelmann, P. K. (1994). Multiple roles and psychological well-being in a national sample of older adults. *Journal of Gerontology: Social Sciences, 49*(6), S277-S285.

Ahmed, F. E. (1992). Effect of nutrition on the health of the elderly. *Journal of the American Dietetic Association, 9,* 1102-1108.

Borges, M. A., Levine, J. R., and Dutton, L. J. (1984). Men's and women's rating of life satisfaction by age of respondent and age interval judged. *Sex Roles, 11,* 3/4.

Bortz, W. M. 11, (1991) *We live too short and die too long.* New York: Bantam Books.

Bosse, R., Aldwin, C. M., Levenson, M. R., Spiro, A. III, & Mroczek, D. K. (1993) Change in social support after retirement: Longitudinal findings from the normative aging study. *Journal of Gerontology: Psychological Sciences, 4*(4), 210-217.

Bulcroft, K. & O'Connor, M. (1986) The importance of dating relationships on quality of life for older persons. *Family Relations, 35,* 397-401.

Caserta, M. S., & Lund, D. A. (1993). Intrapersonal resources and the effectiveness of self-help groups for bereaved older adults. *The Gerontologist, 33*(5), 619629.

Chapuy, M. C., Arlot, M. E., Duboeff, F., Brun, J., Crouzet, B., Arnaud, S., Delmas, P. D., & Meunier, P. J. (1992). Vitamin D3 and calcium to prevent hip fractures in elderly women. *The New England Journal of Medicine, 327*(23), 1637-1642.

Corey, G., (1991) *Theory and practice of counseling and psychotherapy* (4th ed.). Pacific Grove, CA: Brooks/Cole.

Danigelis, N. L., & McIntosh, B., R.N. (1993). Resources and the productive activity of elders: Race and gender as contexts. *Journal of Gerontology: Social Sciences, 48,* S192-S203.

Erikson, E. H., (1959). Psychological *issues: Identity and the life cycle.* New York: International Universities Press, Inc.

Farrell, M. J., Gerontol, M., Gibson, S. J., & Helme; R.D. (1995). The effect of medical status on the activity level of older pain clinic patients. *Journal of the American Geriatrics Society, 43,*102-107.

Grayson, P., Lubin, B., & Van Whitlock, R. (1995). Comparison of depression in the community-dwelling and assisted-living elderly. *Journal of Clinical Psychology, 21,* 18-21.

Hadorn, D. C., & Hays, R. D. (1991). Multitrait-multimethod analysis of health-related quality-of-life measures. *Medical Care, 9,* 829-840.

Hawranik, P., & Walker, J., (1995). Targeting seniors. *Canadian Nurse, August,* 36-39.

Health Insurance Association of America, (1991). Source book of health insurance data. Washington, DC: Author.

Husaini, B. A., & Moore, S. T. (1990). Arthritis disability, depression, and life satisfaction among elderly black people. *Health and Social Work, 15*(4), 253-260.

Statistics Bureau, Management, and Coordination Agency. (1988) *Japan Statistical Yearbook.* Tokyo, Japan: Author.

Keith, P. M., (1986). *Isolation of the unmarried in later life. Family Relations, 35,* 389-395.

Kinney, J. (1991). The elderly. In J. Kinney (Ed.), *Clinical manual of substance abuse* (pp. 233-244), St. Louis, MO: Moseby Year Book.

Kinney, J. & Leaton, G. (1991). *Loosening the grip* (4th ed.). St. Louis, MO: Moseby Year Book.

Lutz, R. W., Pasick, R. J., Pelletier, K. R., & Klehr, L., (1990). Aged to perfection. A prevention program of Department of Mental Health [Brochure].

Manton, K. (1982). Changing concepts of morbidity and mortality in the elderly population. *The Milbank Memorial Fund Quarterly/ Health and Society* 60: 183-244.

Monte, C.F. (1991). *Beneath the mask: An introduction to theories of personality* (4th ed.) Fort Worth, TX: Harcourt Brace.

Neugarten, B. L., Havighurst, R. J., & Tobin, M. A., (1956). The measurement of life satisfaction. *Journal of Gerontology, 16,* 134-143.

Paffenbarger, R. S., Jr., Hyde, R. T., Wing, A. L., Min, I., Jung, D. L., & Kampert, J. B. (1993). The association of changes in physical-activity level and other lifestyle characteristics with mortality among men. *The England Journal of Medicine, 328*(8), 538545.

Roos, P. & Havens, B. (1991). Predictors of successful aging: A twelve year study of Manitoba elderly. *American Journal of Public Health, 1,* 63-67.

Rohm-Young, D., Masaki, K. H., & Curb, D. (1995). Associations of physical activity with performance-based and self-reported physical functioning in older men: The Honolulu heart program. *Journal of the American Geriatrics Society, 43,* 845-854.

Sandvik, L., Erikssen, J., Thaulow, E., Erikssen, G., Mundal, R., & Rodahl, K. (1993). Physical fitness as a predictor of mortality among healthy, middle-aged Norwegian men. *The New England Journal of Medicine, 328*(8), 533-537.

Schmitt, J. P. & Kurdek, L. A., (1985). Age and gender differences in and correlates of loneliness in different relationships. *Journal of Personality Assessments, 5,*485-497.

Shichman, S. & Cooper, E., (1984). Life satisfaction and sex-role concept. *Sex Roles, 11,* 227-240

Simonsick, E. M., Lafferty, M. E., Phillips, C. L., Mendes de Leon, C. F., Kasl, S. V., Seeman, T. E., Fillenbaum, G., Hebert, P., & Lemke, J. H. (1993). Risk due to inactivity in physically capable older adults. *American Journal of Public Health, 10,* 1443-1449.

Steinkamp, M. W. & Kelly, J. R, (1985). Relationships among motivational orientation, level of leisure activity, and life satisfaction in older men and women. *Journal of Psychology, 119,* 509-520.

Strawbridge, W. J., Camacho, T. C., Cohen, R. D., & Kaplan, G. A. (1993). Gender differences in factors associated with change in physical functioning in old age: A 6-year longitudinal study. *The Gerontologist, 11,* 603-609.

Svanborg, A. (1993). A medical-social intervention in a 70 year old Swedish population: Is it possible to postpone functional decline in aging? *Journal of Gerontology, 48,* 84-88.

U. S. Bureau of the Census. (1991). *Population statistics.* U. S. Department of Health and Human Services.

Wolinsky, F. D., Stump, T. E., & Clark, B. 0. (1995). Antecedents and consequences of physical activity and exercise among older adults. *The Gerontologist, 35*, 451-462.

Wolkenstein, A. S. & Butler, D. J. (1992). Quality of life among the elderly: Self-perspectives of some healthy elderly. *Gerontology & Geriatrics Education, 12*(4), 59-68.

2

You Can't Take It With You:
Some Things You Should Do Before You Die

John L. Levy

An essential part of the aging process should be preparing for our dying and death. Unfortunately, many of us practice, with varying degrees of success, the denial that these are ever going to happen to us. In fact, various studies have shown that more than half of American adults do not have a will or other estate plan. Surprisingly, the percentage of wealthy people without such documents is higher than one would expect.

The purpose of this chapter is to encourage readers to face this reality and to make the preparations which will best serve them and those they leave behind. This means facing not just the "practical" issues involved, but also the psychological and spiritual aspects of our dying. I will approach these matters by presenting information and ideas from my own preparations, particularly over the past few years.

Taking up first the practical, here are some recommendations for making advanced preparations

- Ensure that distributions from your estate are as you want them to be and not dictated by the state.
- Minimize problems for survivors—those who will have to make decisions and take actions regarding your belongings and their distribution, especially since they will probably be somewhat emotionally distraught when they must face this challenge.
- Improve the quality of your life from now on.
- Determine whether you have enough assets to support you through the probable rest of your life.

Probably our most important practical task is ensuring that we have in place appropriate legal instructions for the distribution of our assets to the beneficiaries we choose. Often this consists of a Revocable Living Trust. Usually preferable to a stand-alone will, a Revocable Living Trust does not require a probate, as wills do in most states. This type of trust specifies distributions of your estate to the beneficiaries you choose, and names the trustee(s) and successor trustees (in case the named trustee cannot carry out these duties). I have found it important to discuss this in advance with the trustees I would choose, so that it is clear that they are willing to take on these responsibilities. However, it is also possible for the trustee to hire and supervise an attorney or other professional to handle the work.

The trust can specify whatever distributions you wish, including cash, securities, and personal property, and the trustee(s) must carry out these instructions. In almost all cases, I strongly recommend that this document be drawn up, or at least reviewed, by an attorney. Where the estate or its distribution is complex, or where there is any likelihood of controversy among heirs, a lawyer who specializes in estate planning would be the best choice.

A Living Trust does not include funds in a retirement account. Distribution of these upon your death is specified in Beneficiary Forms provided by the funds in which your retirement accounts are invested, and for each of these you need to specify your primary beneficiary and contingent beneficiaries, those who will inherit your retirement funds if your primary beneficiary(ies) are not living. Distributions from your retirement accounts to your spouse are not treated as her taxable income until the time of withdrawal. IRA distributions to anyone else are taxed as income when they are received, so most people make their spouses the primary beneficiaries of their retirement accounts.

Both your living trust and retirement account beneficiary forms should be reviewed every year or so to ensure that they still reflect your wishes. I and others I know often find ourselves confronting resistance to looking at all this again, and we need motivation and self-discipline to face this rather daunting task regularly. I have known a number of families, especially those with significant wealth, who have held one or more meetings of all concerned family members to discuss distribution of their estate. You may want to begin by telling them, perhaps in writing, the essential elements of your current estate plan, making clear that you welcome their input and are open to making changes if this seems right. If your estate is large and/or complex, you should instruct your estate planning attorney to provide a brief summary of its provisions in plain, easily understood language. Where there is likely to be conflict within the group, many families have brought in an outside mediator/consultant to help with this and make sure that everyone present is heard. This is a role I have assumed with a number of wealthy families, and have learned that the presence of a neutral facilitator can increase the comfort of those involved and help them to be more open and honest with one another.

Where applicable, your living trust should specify who will take responsibility for your children who are minors. Naturally, you will need to discuss this with those named and be sure that they are willing to accept these responsibilities. You will also need to discuss this decision with the affected children, if they are old enough to understand what it will mean.

Where the funds to be passed on are large, and/or if you have strong philanthropic inclinations, there are also various charitable trusts and/or bequests you can set up with the help of a planned-giving specialist who understands them and how they might be of value in your individual case. Planned Giving Consultants, community foundations, and some estate planning attorneys offer these services. Philanthropic trusts can offer significant savings in income and estate taxes, especially for large estates. If you choose to use one of these, it is important that your heirs know about it in advance, understand your reasons for doing so, and know how this will affect their inheritances.

A very valuable gift, but one we usually do not think to give, is a letter to each of your survivors, providing detailed information that will be helpful to them when you die. This is not an easy thing to do, but I and others have found it both gratifying and instructive. To write such a letter, I suggest you imagine yourself in the survivor's place and jot down all the things you would need to know in order to do what you have been instructed to do. The information below is based upon what I included in my own letter.

- Information about the location of important papers, such as the living trust (which some of them should already have), recent tax returns, insurance documents, professional papers, important personal correspondence, etc.
- Instructions or suggestions about what to do with these about the distribution of your possessions—home, furnishings, automobile(s), art objects, clothing, music and video, photographs, etc. Indicate who you want to receive certain objects, especially those with significant monetary or emotional value, suggest how to make decisions on others, what to do with those none of them wants. In doing this, it is important to keep in mind perceived fairness, to avoid dissension and disappointment.

- Locations of a safety deposit box, its key, and other vaults. Who has authority to enter it?
- Information about the approximate value of your estate now, with strongly stressed caveats about how this may change, especially if you will need to pay for your own or others' illnesses later on. Indicate briefly how your trust distributes your assets now, with explanations as appropriate. Make it clear, however, that any of your instructions can be changed, and that you are inviting their questions and suggestions. You may want to set up a meeting of all involved to discuss all this, particularly if they want to do so. My professional experience has taught me that heirs do not like surprises, and often feel disappointed, resentful, and even litigious toward both the deceased and their fellow heirs.
- Details about your wishes as to funeral arrangements, disposition of your remains, and funeral or memorial service. A sincere expression of your affection for and appreciation of those you are leaving behind. This can mean a lot to them both now and later, and you will find the experience of writing these words most rewarding.

I encourage you to review this letter fairly often, as you are likely to find you want to make changes, and then distribute the revised letter to those involved. I have done this every year or so, and, by the way, it is a lot easier to rewrite all this now than it was to write it from scratch first time.

There are pamphlets available from several hospice organizations providing information on these and other issues. You may even want to discuss some of these issues with local hospice staff.

Now let me turn to the psychological and spiritual issues related to death and dying. There are a number of good reasons for dealing with these well ahead of time:

- To ameliorate the anxiety and depression which almost always accompany the realization that death is imminent.
- To make the dying experience optimal for ourselves, for those who care about us, and for those who will be our final caretakers.
- To enable us to be more helpful to those we love who are dying before we do.
- To prepare as best we can for whatever we may experience after our deaths.

Deciding and communicating our desires regarding the circumstances of our dying is most important. Where do we want to die? I recommend that, if feasible, this not be in a hospital, since medical responsibilities usually interfere with the atmosphere we are likely to want as we are dying. Whom do we wish to have present during our last illness, dying, and death? What spiritual surroundings and support, if any, do we wish? Do we want a counselor, clergy or other spiritual professional present? Photographs or art work? Special music? Meaningful texts read to us? What else? I have included all this in my own letter to my wife and survivors.

It is most important that we make *very* clear our desires and intentions regarding the circumstances of our dying. This includes filling out and distributing several documents:

- **Instructions for Health Care:** This document lets you state your wishes about medical care when you can no longer speak for yourself. It makes specific your intentions regarding treatment when your death is imminent and medical care can only prolong your life, often rather briefly, but not save it, or when your level of consciousness is such that continuing to live seems not worthwhile.
- **Durable Power of Attorney for Health Care:** This document names someone(s) to make decisions about your medical care when you are no longer able to do so, and supplements the instructions described above.
- **Donations of Organs at Death (optional):** This document states your wishes, if any, regarding organ donation.

All three documents must be witnessed by two people and/or a notary public in order to be effective.

The information stated above comes from a very valuable document, the Advance Healthcare Directive, prepared and distributed by Compassion and Choices, a fine non-profit organization focused on enabling people to die as they wish. You can download all these materials from their website, www.compassionandchoices.org, or write them at PO Box 101810, Denver, CO 80250-1810. Requirements about the structure and content of these forms vary from state to state, so you will have to indicate which state you plan to use them in.

In regard to the process of dying, a good deal of information and counsel is available, as well as books, articles, videos, etc., many but not all from various spiritual traditions. Some books I and others have found helpful in preparing for the dying experience include:

- *The Grace in Dying* by Kathleen Dowling Singh (2000)
- *Who Dies?* by Stephen and Ondrea Levine (1989)
- *Advice on Dying (and living a better life)* by the Dalai Lama (Gyatso, 2002)
- *The Tibetan Book of Living and Dying* by Sogyal Rinpoche (1992)
- *Graceful Passages: A Companion for Living and Dying*, a book and CD produced by Michael Stillwater and Gary Malkin (2006)

Hospice organizations have been developing and growing all over the country for several decades now. Their staff and volunteers provide psychical and emotional support and care there for terminally ill people and their families. Besides being present for the dying person, they are trained to be there for those being left behind, during and after the death of a loved one. They offer advice and instructions for caring for the dying person as well as emotional support for those dealing with the expectation and the actuality of the loved one's death. Their compassionate support can also be helpful to family members preparing for their own deaths.

Hospice workers provide assistance with the physical aspects of dying, including measures to reduce physical and psychological pain. Some, but not all, focus as well on spiritual aspects of the dying process, and you may want to know in advance who these are.

This chapter has been based on my own searching and concerns. I have tried to cover the issues involved as I understand them, and to provide useful information regarding these. I know that as you look into these matters for yourself, you will form your own ideas about them and find your own information and resources. However, my principal, heartfelt message here is universal: DON'T PUT IT OFF! Death is not just for others. It is going to come to you and those you love, and the more you are able to accept and prepare for it well ahead of time, the better the remainder of your life.

References

Gyatso, T. (2002). *Advice on dying and living a better life* (Ed. & Trans. by J. Hopkins). New York: Atria Books.

Levine, S. & Levine, O. (1989). *Who dies? An investigation of conscious living and conscious dying.* Garden City, NY: Anchor.

Rinpoche, S. (1992). *The Tibetan book of living and dying.* San Francisco: Harper.

Singh, K. D. (2000). *The grace in dying: How we are transformed spiritually as we die.* San Francisco: HarperOne.

Stillwater, M. & Malkin, G. (2006). *Graceful passages: A companion for living and dying* (2nd ed.). Plymouth, MN: New World Library.

3

Speak from the Heart

Will Rogers

As an attorney, one of the most meaningful aspects of my work occurs when a client asks me to assist him or her in creating an estate plan.[1] Sometimes the quality of the exchange that I have with someone engaged in such a process can enter the domain of the sacred.

Many times a person is prompted to create a will because he or she is on the verge of a long trip or an anticipated hospitalization. Under such circumstances I gather information quickly, sometimes over the telephone, and the end product is usually the standard, efficient, dry document that simply states who gets what.

However, when a person is not under any outward pressure to create a will and, rather than rushing through the process, takes the time necessary to think deeply about his or her inevitable demise, the end product can be something of deep significance and meaning for those left behind as well as for the person creating the will.

In addition to creating a will, there is a long tradition, especially strong within Judaism, of creating a document referred to as an "ethical will." An ethical will is a testamentary document that does not dispose of things; rather, it is intended to leave something of greater value: words of wisdom from the accumulation of a lifetime of experiences. It is an attempt to give something of the heart, to impart values, to share the lessons learned by suffering and love, to give words of forgiveness, faith, and courage.

In pondering all that is involved in creating an estate plan that disposes of assets, the thought of death is always lurking just outside the door. Most struggle to keep the door tightly closed. Contemplating the creation of an ethical will opens the door and welcomes the thought of death. When the shadow of death is welcomed with joy and curiosity, as a student welcoming a beloved teacher, perspectives change. Fully present to the knowledge of the transitory nature of life, a person sees her or his past, present, and future in a new light. The present becomes pregnant with meaning and significance. Decisions regarding how the remaining moments–moments blithely assumed to remain–are informed by the awareness that the foothold on the planet is indeed precarious.

The author of an ethical will sees the so-called failures and mistakes of the past as valuable, hard-won lessons, lessons that have led to wisdom, wisdom worthy of memorializing in print for future generations. His or her life's story becomes a page to be inserted in the Book of Life, to be read even by those not yet born.

The tradition of creating an ethical will is alive and well and is getting more and more attention. Many books and articles are available for those interested in this subject. Perhaps the best book is *So That Your Values Live On: Ethical Wills and How to Prepare Them*, by Riemer and Stamper (1991). Riemer's book contains many beautiful and touching ethical wills created in the last two centuries by rabbis and lay persons. I have included an excerpt below, a brief introduction from an ethical will written by an American in 1951. Following that, I have included the introduction in my own ethical will written about 15 years ago to my son, although at the time I had no knowledge of the tradition of ethical wills. I hope that these passages convey some of the flavor of what such a document can contain.

Dear Children:

Somewhere among these papers is a will made out by a lawyer. Its purpose is to dispose of any material things which I may possess at the time of my departure from this world to the unknown adventure beyond.

I hope its terms will cause no ill will among you. It seemed sensible when I made it. After all, it refers only to material things which we enjoy only temporarily.

I am more concerned with having you inherit something that is vastly more important. (Riemer & Stamper, 1991, p. 125)

The writer continues with a bit of philosophy, some requests ("care for your mother"), some exhortations ("carry your Jewish heritage with dignity"), expressions of regret for careless words, and a touching ending that brought tears to my eyes.

Here is the introduction to my ethical will:

For My Beloved Son:

As I write this on July 3, 1993, you are but 3 1/2 months old and I am a few days shy of my birthday.

Life in this world is uncertain, change is the only constant. It is my deepest wish to accompany you as you navigate the many twists and turns the path of life will present you. But I might not be present with you in a physical sense. We may never meet as adults; we have had delightful conversations together, but we may never have a conversation that we both fully comprehend; hence this letter.

This letter is to serve as my last testament, a document in which I wish to convey all the wisdom and love that I wished I had imparted to you in person. This is a daunting and impossible task, for nothing I write will ever substitute for a loving glance from papa when you need reassurance or forgiveness, and nothing will substitute for a word of wisdom from papa when you are confused and feel lost. However, if we are parted, this is the only medium God will grant for the communication of what I wish to impart.

Then in about a page and a half I attempt to share some of my insights, advice, and words of wisdom. Even though my son is now 15, I have not revised the document as I consider it an accurate expression of my truth at the time I wrote it. I plan to add to it, but not rewrite it.

There is sufficient information available to attorneys on how to guide a client in the creation of a will and of an ethical will. However, some people need something more. Some need to commune, face to face, in order to share the contents of their hearts. In contrast to the information available on creating ethical wills, I have found no information for attorneys on how to assist the elderly or dying in going beneath the surface of the "who gets what," in order to step into the deeper realms of meaningfulness. This is the purpose of the present article.

I write with the hope of conveying something of value to all those who work with the elderly or the dying. I confess that I have had no training as a psychologist and no training in working with the dying. I can attest that I have been deeply engaged in a spiritual tradition for the past 35 years, and that my "method," such as it is, continues to be informed by my own inner journey. I assume that there are professionals much more knowledgeable than I about this subject. I am writing from my own experience, with all its assorted limitations.

Some clients need nothing more than a patient listener. I once sat with a woman for almost six hours as she poured out her story of 86 years. All I had to do was be present. As I sat with her in her tiny one-room poverty-hotel room, I heard a tale of how she achieved fame and wealth, of how she lost fame and wealth, of having family and friends, and of losing family and friends. It was a tale of love and suffering. A few times she paused self-consciously and said, "Oh my! I never told this story to anyone." I felt privileged to be the recipient of secrets that had never been given voice.

Most people need more assistance. Therefore, when a client wants to create a will, I approach our meeting with great delicacy. I know that some people have navigated many barriers just to get to our first meeting. Some clients have never met with an attorney before and are nervous; some have had to sort through complex and painful family relationships; some have worried about the costs of a professionally drafted will; some have overcome the superstition that creating a will is an omen that they are about to die; some are perhaps facing their fear of death for the first time.

I prepare by inwardly removing any barriers that tend to accrue to the attorney in an attorney-client relationship, including the stereotypical attorney persona and the professional and emotional distance that some attorneys foster. I enter into my heart and, silently, welcome the person as a human being, a person of infinite complexity and mystery.

I usually begin the meeting by reminding the person that everything he or she tells me is completely confidential, that I will carry what is told to me to my grave. As we converse I try to be completely and utterly present to the other person. I listen intently. I respond with tact and consideration.

I let the person know that I have no judgments about his or her decisions and that I am standing outside of a unique family history, and the associated baggage, that may be burdening her or him. I try to give an honest reflection of what I hear. And the only way I know of conveying a nonjudgmental attitude is to really *be* nonjudgmental. I cannot fake it. I must be sincere. I become completely accepting.

The meeting is fluid. Sometimes a person really wants or needs me to tell them what they should do. I then shift from being a sympathetic friend into the role of an attorney. My voice and demeanor may change as I speak with authority, with *gravitas,* giving advice or reassurance.

However, it I sense that the person wants to tell me something of a sensitive nature, something that may be difficult to express, I may ask a question to give the person an opening. Sometimes, there is no opening and the person just wants to share personal wishes about the designation of his or her property after death.

Sometimes when I provide an opening, a burden carried for years comes to the surface. A person may tell me of his or her estrangement from a child, a failure in business, a deep longing unfulfilled, or a lapse in moral judgment with disastrous consequences.

I might then become a father-confessor hearing of sins long kept hidden. The person might be crying or barely holding back tears. Perhaps I see before me an elderly man or woman nearing the end of life, and acutely aware the end is near, and yet I may hear a story of a burden that seems to have no end. A few words can be the window into a pain held for decades.

At this point, I may want to simply become a witness and marvel at the privilege of seeing into the private life of another. At such times, I would like to remain silent and simply hold the moment with my loving attention. However, I am an attorney and I have assumed a different role than that of a compassionate, silent witness. The word "attorney" comes from the Old French *atorne*, "one appointed." Rightly or wrongly, I assume that the Universe, in its infinite wisdom, has appointed me to speak in such a tender and significant moment.

What do I say? I speak from my heart, with simple words, very rarely giving advice, and always with great trepidation, knowing that my words may be a part of the *denouement* of an entire life story. I try to draw the words from the well of wisdom that I have touched on my own very personal journey into life's deepest mysteries. I rarely quote scriptures or the words from any religious figure, as such words might have huge negative associations. For some, the word "God" is a word charged with disagreeable associations.

However, sometimes I do use religious words when I know that a person is deeply engaged in a particular religious tradition. I created a will for my uncle as he was dying. The process involved several visits to his bedside over the course of several days. He was surrounded by relatives afraid to speak the words "death" or "dying" in his presence. They assured my uncle that he was going to be okay. I knew he was dying and I knew that he knew it. I also knew that he was a devout Catholic. At the end of the process, moments after signing his will, I said to him, "Now Uncle Al, you can go and be with Jesus." He thanked me with tears in his eyes. I felt a burden lift from the room. He died a few hours later. Psychologists have told me that I gave him permission to die. Even though I did not share my uncle's religion, my words were sincere and sincerely spoken.

In general when I am with someone nearing the end, I look the person in the eyes when I speak. I touch his or her hand or arm, if appropriate. I speak plainly and slowly using short and concise sentences. I might be as brief as, "You did the best you could," or "there is nothing more for you to do." And if said with sincerity, it might be enough.

On rare occasions, I may interject some of my own personal journey, especially my missteps. When I share the story of some action that I regret, or when I reveal a bit of my own woundedness, I do so with the intent of making the other person more at ease in sharing something from his or her own depths.

Those of us who have the privilege to work with the elderly or the dying, whether as an attorney, healthcare professional, hospice worker, caretaker, son, daughter, friend, or spouse, can provide services of profound meaningfulness. The more we are conscious of the privilege of service to the elderly or dying, the more we can play a significant role in the cosmic drama of life and death.

References

Riemer, J. & Stamper, N. (1991). *So that your values live on: Ethical wills and how to prepare them*. Woodstock, VT: Jewish Lights Publishing.

Part 2

Gifts Returned:
The Mind and Body

4

Aging and Neurocognition

Gregg Richardson

I am now 60, have spent the past ten years as a full-time clinical neuropsychologist for Kaiser Permanente, and cared for both my parents in my Berkeley home from 1997 to 2005 (Dad) and 2007 (Mom), coordinating their medical and home care and managing their finances. After Mom came home from a skilled nursing facility in late 2004, I tried caring for her myself, but within two weeks had hired a weekday caretaker. I quickly realized how draining it is to add hours of caregiving to a full-time work schedule, and suddenly appreciated the burdens carried by single working parents.

My favorite joke of last year was about the older man who walks into a bar, goes up to an attractive woman on a bar stool and says, "Hi. Do I come here often?" The older you are, the more likely you are to appreciate that joke, since we all get more forgetful as we age. In fact, memory is only one of the areas in which we can decline as we age. My mother's physician once sent her home with a list of the things that can happen as we get older. The one I immediately understood read, "You know you're over 50 when an 'all-nighter' means not getting up to pee." That is in part because our bladders lose some of their elasticity with age and become less "forgiving" if we drink a lot of liquid. It is why many older people don't drink much after dinner or before a long car or airplane ride.

We neuropsychologists think in terms of "domains," that is, areas of cognitive functioning. There is mild disagreement about how many of these there are, but most agree on the following skill areas: Attention, Language, Visuospatial, Motor, Memory, and Executive Function. As a neuropsychologist, I assess these areas of brain function in people who have (or are afraid they have) suffered damage from Alzheimer's (one form of dementia), strokes, accidents, Parkinson's disease, Huntington's disease, exposure to toxic substances, meningitis, and other conditions. My patients include Blacks who came out of the

South during World War II to work in Henry Kaiser's shipyards and other businesses here in California; Whites who were born here or have immigrated from around the world, often to study or teach at the University of California, Berkeley; Latinos who have multi-century family histories in California or who came here recently; Asians from many countries with old or recent family histories in California; and just about every other sort of person in every category you can imagine. Most, although not all, are older, with normal problems due only to normal aging. I am usually able to look my patients in the eye and say, "You don't have Alzheimer's. You're just 65 (or 45 or 85)." I also see younger people who have suffered head injuries in motorcycle and other accidents, survived meningitis or encephalitis or other diseases, or fear that they have adult Attention Deficit Hyperactivity Disorder (ADHD).

Many of my older patients are not aging normally, however, and I often have to tell them (and the spouse or child who has accompanied them) that their condition is more serious. In such situations humor can be useful, but I have to use it carefully. It is good to be able to laugh about our mortality—about aging, disease, and death—but I need to be reasonably certain that the patient is able to share in the laughter before I attempt to evoke it. Compassion and sensitivity are essential. They help me provide better care to my patients and make caregiving easier on me. Still, the realities of aging, disease, and death are not altered. The mortality factors always remain, however we feel about them and whatever sort of spiritual support we cultivate for ourselves. Death is the free space on our life's bingo cards.

What I want to do here is to present something like a case history of my parents, discussing their medical and cognitive problems and their ultimately easy deaths, and then talk about each of the neurocognitive domains listed above in terms of how these were affected by changes in my parents' brains or bodies, and how those changes affected them in practical ways.

So let me first say a little more about both my long-term patients, that is, my parents, who are now both deceased. I brought them out here in 1997 because they could no longer live alone in Mount Healthy, Ohio. Yes, you read correctly. It is now part of the sprawl of Cincinnati, but was much more distinctly small-town when I was young. Mom's family has been there for 10 generations, so I had her and Dad visit me a few times over several years to get to know my home and the Bay Area generally. Then, one night on the phone I asked, "Would you consider moving out here?" It only took a few seconds for Mom to say, "Well, yes, we could do that," so I knew that they had certainly discussed the whole thing, because leaving their home of 50 years and all her family and their neighbors had to have been a huge decision. I, in truth, hesitated to take them out of that network, because I knew they would be leaving a broad, long-time, and wonderful support system behind. On the other hand, all the neighbors were about as old as they were and were very happy to see them move out and live with me because they knew that, as neighbors, they were not going to be able to care for Mom and Dad themselves. I still get teary when I remember the morning we left our old home, the home I grew up in, at dawn, with all my parents' things in a U-Haul. All the neighbors were either at their windows or in their yards waving us off and shouting goodbyes in the gray early light until we were out of sight. Those who are still alive keep in touch, and repeatedly assure me that we made the right decision in leaving because "Mount Healthy is just not the same anymore." Still I know they miss having Mom and Dad among them.

So Dad lived for eight years here, and Mom for ten. She came out here with a left hip replacement and Dad with a history of TIAs, those little mini-strokes. After moving here Dad had two moderate strokes; Mom had one stroke, a right total-knee replacement, and at 80 a broken right hip and femur sustained in a fall, necessitating surgery and a long convalescence that basically left her unable to walk much afterward, leading finally to the home care I mentioned above. I still cared for her on weekends and holidays, however, and found myself coming home earlier and traveling less as a result. As Dad aged he had increasing difficulty walking, and became more forgetful, confused, and irritable. All in all, the slope of their decline was not too steep for the first seven years, but then became noticeably steeper. It was like bricks had been coming out of their foundations here and there, now and then, and suddenly I realized how unstable their structures had become, how increasingly vulnerable to total collapse.

I highly recommend reading Sherwin Nuland's (1995) book, *How We Die.* He is a physician who talks in his book about the various things that take us out in the end, how the body's systems interact, and how weakening one system weakens the others; it is a very straightforward and somewhat frightening book if you are still young and healthy, but also very compassionate and humane. It is also a wonderful inoculation, giving us a chance to consider the specifics of aging in the relative comfort of our minds before we must confront them in our own or others' bodies. I have come to think it a great gift to be able to reflect on my own (and others') declines and deaths beforehand.

So now let me focus more specifically on my parents, beginning with patient Marian, my mother, who lived in my little retirement home in Berkeley, California, for ten years. She was pretty cognitively sound and in reasonable health from the time she came here in April of 1997 until August of 2003, when she suffered a mild stroke, then began falling, and finally broke her right hip/leg in that fall in November of 2004. We also learned after her 2003 stroke that she was in chronic right heart failure, that the valve on the right side of the heart was sort of tattered, so that about a third of the blood that got pumped up to the top chamber was falling right back down into the lower chamber. So the right heart responded by working harder and getting ever larger, and it could only do that for so long before it wore out. That was the loosest brick in her foundation. And secondary to that, the blood was not getting drained from her liver very well, which meant her blood was not very clean and that meant, third, that her brain was not getting the best quality blood all the time, leading to a "transient encephalopathy," which means she seemed demented at times, forgetting where she was, and what she had just done, and confusing my name with Dad's. To return to my earlier analogy, she now had a loose brick in the attic as well.

Now let me go back to that stroke in August of 2003. It was in her right hemisphere, with resulting left-sided weakness and numbness. Mother of a neuropsychologist, she knew enough on the day it happened to recognize it; she had bent down to pick something up, realized first that she could not grasp it, and then that she could not stand on her left leg. We had a housemate at that time who happened to be at home. She had him call my cell phone and describe her symptoms. I told him to call 911 and explain to the operator that an 80-year-old woman just had a stroke. I arrived home while the EMTs were all still there, and they took great care of her in the ambulance and in hospital.[1]

After she recovered and returned home we did not notice any particular physical problems, apart from the fact that she just seemed a little weaker in the legs. But then I began to notice more subtle changes. One was that she began losing her time/date stamp, that is, she often no longer knew what day or time it was, or even whether it was morning or night. This is a very good example of how, when we have some kind of damage to the brain, we can lose abilities that we have always just taken for granted. It would not occur to us to think that we would not

---

[1] I showed up at the emergency room wearing my own Kaiser ID; I'm sure they would have given her good care even without that, but at the time I was taking no chances.

know the day of the week or the approximate time of day. Aging, in other words, is often not just a vague decline into wrinkles, weakness, forgetfulness, and the need to get up to pee at night, but often involves very specific losses that we would never have guessed beforehand.

The other thing Mom lost after that stroke was her sense of place familiarity; she became convinced at times that although our house looked the same, it really was not ours, that we were living in a sort of phantom home that was a copy of our true one. This experience was mixed with confusion about our neighbors and surroundings, in which she would confuse our current neighbors and their homes with those from back in Mount Healthy, or imagine that we were actually living in the house of a friend, near either our old Mount Healthy home or our current California home. There's a name for this condition, Capgras Syndrome, but the essential point is to understand that our sense of familiarity can be detached from things, that formerly familiar things and people and places can become unfamiliar, or unfamiliar ones familiar (a different syndrome). Put another way, the sense of "familiarity" we take for granted can actually become separated from our daily thoughts and experiences.

One day she was convinced that a friend's kitchen was like the one in the "jail," the jail being her hospital room after that fall, where they had her in restraints because she was trying to get out of bed with a broken hip. I had just returned from a neuropsychology conference in Seattle—I was literally just off the plane—and the hospital staff called and said, "Your mother's screaming. We can't settle her down." I asked them to give her the phone and she said, "They're holding me in jail and they won't let me go and these people are crazy" but I was able to calm her by saying, repeatedly, "No, Mom, you're in the hospital and you've broken your hip and you mustn't get out of bed." Later she remembered this episode and was able to laugh about it. I consciously and wherever possible used the strategies of normalizing her experiences and getting her to laugh about things she could not change. I might say, "You know, Mom, you don't have to go to work, so what does it matter what day it is?" or, "Don't worry about the time. We'll tell you what time it is if you want to know." I made it a rule never to say, "I just told you that," instead answering her questions afresh each time, and this helped to keep unnecessary anxiety from building up and making things worse.

Mom was a woman with several specific but related losses—her heart affecting her liver, which in turn was affecting her brain; direct brain damage from her strokes; weakness in her legs; specific cognitive losses. We were just sort of waiting to see what was going to give out next, and at one point I told her outright, "You're probably going to go to bed some night and just not wake up." We agreed that this would be wonderful, because she was not in any great discomfort and there was no serious and painful disease threatening her apart from arthritis. She was probably just going to stop without much warning, and what a lovely way to go. This is a woman whose grandmother said just before her 90th birthday, "Ninety's too old. I've had enough, my friends are all dead, and it's time to go." There was nothing really wrong with her that anybody knew of. She just went to bed and three days later she was gone. I have always hoped I will have the awareness and courage to do that when the time comes, but I have my doubts, both about my own capability to carry out such a plan and about what today's medical-legal system will allow.

In the end, Mom became increasingly anxious while alone at home during the day (the caretaker came to "package" her in the morning and evening). One day she managed to descend two flights of stairs and wander across the street, without her walker. Neighbors responded quickly, took her home, and called me. Soon after this I found her a very pleasant, clean, and friendly board and care home (six residents and two full-time caregivers) very close to where we lived. We got her to move by responding to her frequent question, "When are we going home?" with "Now!," bundling her into the car, and taking her to her new room, which we had prepared ahead of time. She was only slightly confused and quickly responded to the kindness of the Taiwanese man who was to be her primary caretaker. To illustrate how far her language skills had deteriorated at that point, she never realized that this caretaker spoke virtually no English; she would chat with him and introduce him (repeatedly) as if nothing were out of the ordinary, and also enjoyed watching Taiwanese television programs with him![2]

After slightly more than three months, the staff called me to say that Mom was not well and had gone to bed. She said she was in no pain, laughed often but could not explain why, and died in her sleep two days later. I had been with her until very near the end, then returned to deal with all the final details (police, her physician, the coroner) before the woman who came to take her to the University of California San Francisco Medical School was allowed to do so (we had all donated our bodies to science when we wrote up our wills and other final documents shortly after they came to stay with me).

---

[2] Unfamiliar with different Asian ethnicities, she at one point announced that she had just gotten back from Japan, having confused TV with reality. I responded that it was wonderful that she could travel so cheaply, a joke that went right over her head.

Dad had died two years earlier, after an intervention radiologist had precipitated a third and final stroke after threading a catheter from his femoral artery up into his brain and squirting into the arterioles around one of his left sinus cavities something to stop chronic bleeding. This periodic bleeding had gone on for months, even after the removal of some sinus polyps and several visits to the ER. Dad was enthusiastic about the catheter procedure—as a former tool and die maker he could visualize it and thought it made sense—even though he said he understood the risks to him after two strokes. Late that night, it became clear that the catheter had knocked something loose on its journey upwards and that Dad had suffered a third stroke. The staff seemed to think he would recover, but he did not agree and tried, as I reflect back on it, to convey to me his awareness that this was the end. Within 48 hours he had slipped into a coma, and after a meeting with hospital staff to review his final directives and Mom's and my wishes, we agreed to remove his feeding tube. After ten days of "comfort care"—morphine, hydration, daily washing, clean linens—he died so quietly that no one realized it until a nurse came in to check on him. His body, like Mom's, went off to the UCSF Medical School. We had watched his dementia progress over the previous few years, with more forgetfulness, an inability to track woodcarving or clock repair projects (he would start these, then forget what he had already done and not know what to do next), confusion about his medications (I finally took over management of these), and greater irritability, including anger when he could not follow a conversation or believed we were stealing things he had simply misplaced. All this was in addition to chronic knee and back pain. So his end was welcome and the cause of it something of a surprise.

We held a potluck memorial at home. Fifty people came—old friends of mine who had known him over the last nine years , old friends of his from his woodcarving group, a woman he had known and often eaten with from the McDonald's in downtown Berkeley (Mom was convinced at moments that they were having a secret affair)—and we all ate and talked and reminisced. He would have enjoyed it much more than a funeral. Within six months I had managed to clean up his side of the bedroom and replace all his things with a single photo on the night table. Over the remaining months of her life at home, Mom would still reach over at night to find and hold his hand, still real in her mind after nearly 63 years of marriage; she would also hear his voice at times or see him sitting in their love seat in the TV room. After years of repetition, internal memories can become external realities as dementia weakens the barrier between the internal and external worlds.

A big lesson here for me here was that after years of wondering and worrying how we will die, we often end up surprised. The Grim Reaper had come in the guise of a nosebleed rather an accident, a heart attack, or a cancer, and all those years of worry had been for nothing, time that could have been better spent planning useful things, focusing on loved ones, enjoying life while it lasted. I now live with the knowledge that I am most likely to be taken out by something cardiovascular and focus instead on enjoying the people and pets and activities I love, a change in attitude for which I thank Dad.

Lessons on the Neurocognitive Domains

So that is my case presentation, an interesting but not unusual one, with a typical blend of physiological and cognitive changes due to aging. Now let me speak more specifically about the neurocognitive domains I listed above, using my parents as examples where possible.

Attention/Concentration. These refer to your ability to simply focus on something and then to keep your focus on it until some goal has been accomplished, such as completing four pages of written text, planting a row of tomatoes, reading a magazine article, or carving the head of a horse and leaving the body for later. How well can you count backward from 20 to 1 or keep subtracting 7s from 100? Such tasks are specific, and I can use them to test you and then compare your performance to the performances of others. Even without formal tests, I was able to observe how well and for how long my parents could persist at a task, such as reading the newspaper or washing the dishes, before their mind (or body) wandered off. Mom was pretty good at focusing, especially on reading, and not easily distracted until the last year or two of her life. Dad tended to get confused and distracted more easily during his last years, both by external stimuli and by his emotional reactions to things. He also had problems doing two things at once, like watching TV and having a conversation; *divided attention* is often difficult for the elderly.

Language skills. Do you understand what others are saying? Are you able to respond to them coherently? Are you able to comprehend what you read? Can you still write a coherent letter, find words easily in conversation, or name objects or pictures of them? How quickly can you produce words in a category, such as the names of fruits or animals? Both my parents wrote and read well, although arthritis affected Mom's handwriting toward the end and she tended to do less of it as a result, meaning fewer letters home, fewer Christmas cards, and an end to the daily notes she had made on calendars about what she and Dad had done each day and where and how every penny was spent, a habit going back to the beginning of their marriage in 1941. They had no problems with oral skills—comprehension and expression—but both developed trouble finding words at times. As a result, Mom came to use "he" and "she" when she couldn't think of someone's name (e.g., "She brought those lemons," referring to our neighbor), hoping I would know who she meant from context. Dad would become angry, when describing recent events, if I did not know what "the thing" referred to.

Visuospatial skills. These often get lost without anyone noticing. If you are well-spoken and remember who people are, they will assume you are cognitively intact. But you can be very well-spoken and still have lost the ability to understand a diagram or map or to interpret letters on a page, and this will be less obvious to others and to you, or perhaps mistakenly attributed to memory loss. You may have trouble finding things at home, not just because your memory is poorer but because you are not making sense of what you see; you put something down out of motor habit but don't take that little mental snapshot of it sitting there on the once-familiar kitchen counter. And who will notice this if you live alone or with a spouse who does the same thing? You put something down, then no longer fully recognize it or its surroundings, and where did it go? Maybe it's a document you need at tax time or a bill that needs paying, and you can't find it. And such visuospatial loss is just as real as a language deficit and can significantly affect your life, but it tends not to be seen unless someone is testing you for it or it has caused a significant problem. Often such problems are not noticed until you start wandering off or getting lost.

Motor skills. Can you translate my words into actions? Can you, at my verbal request, wave to me, or pretend to pour coffee into a cup, add sugar, and stir it? Can you do these things in proper order? Can you learn a sequence of hand positions or tie your shoes? Abilities like these can also be lost even though you still speak well and do not appear particularly forgetful. Mom's and Dad's *neurocognitive* motor skills were okay up until the end, although arthritis and surgical procedures over the years had reduced their manual dexterity, agility and range of motion (leading, in fact, to the fall that broke Mom's hip).

Memory skills. These are the ones we hear most about, and their loss is part of a dementia diagnosis, but they can be lost in different ways. You can lose verbal memory—what was on the shopping list I did not bring with me to the market? What was it you told me not to forget this morning?—but you can also lose visual memory, perhaps not remembering a new face or a familiar place. You can also lose motor memory, forgetting how to sequence tasks—preparing that cup of coffee, tying a necktie (do you remember neckties?), dancing steps you used to perform without thinking.

There are visual and verbal and motor memory *modalities*, and short-term and long-term memories, and other ways to divide memory up, and my job is to find out which of these, if any, has been impaired. Very often, I will have people with fine verbal memories, but impaired visual memories. Mom became somewhat more forgetful visually, mostly forgetting where she had put things, but as I said earlier, her stroke had also affected her sense of place familiarity, and she also had a lifelong difficulty with map-reading, so these problems interacted. In addition, she could no longer keep track of all the news clippings she used to save—this was an obsessive-compulsive behavior related to lifelong anxiety—and led to piles of paper all over our Mount Healthy house, hundreds of pounds of paper that had to be left behind when we moved. Once in California, I set limits on what she could save, and as it became increasingly clear that once she had bagged something she never looked at it again. I confess that I made the decision to recycle the third oldest bag whenever she had filled two new ones. She did not realize I was doing it (or at least never said so), so what was the harm? Dad was somewhat forgetful of both conversations and of where he had put things, and was more prone to anger and suspicion, so he often complained that we had moved or stolen things from him (after his death I found these things behind other objects in his room; he had covered them up but not recalled doing so), and also complained at times that we were lying about having told him things earlier.

Executive functions. If someone has frontal brain damage from an accident or stroke or *frontotemporal dementia* (a type different from Alzheimer's), she or he is more likely to display losses in this domain. Executive skills have to do with planning, organizing, carrying out, and evaluating tasks. I might ask a woman patient (or her spouse), for example, "When was the last time you threw a dinner party?" and if she answers, "Oh, I haven't done that in years," I will inquire further to find out if this is situational—that her friends are all dead or unable to get out, or that she is living in a senior efficiency apartment—or if the tasks of making a guest list, calling people, shopping, preparing a meal, and cleaning up are just too much for her now. Mom tended to feel overwhelmed by parties at the house, so I usually kept them small and gave her just one or two tasks to complete, like baking her famous brownies (while she still could) or deciding which dishes did not belong to us and needed to be returned to those who had left them behind. This made her feel useful but not overwhelmed. Or I might ask a male patient if he has hobbies and when he completed his last project. My father was very handy, a tool and die maker all his working life and an amateur woodcarver in his later years, but in the end he was overwhelmed by even small projects, like carving a small duck. I still have projects in the garage that he started but never finished due to his inability to hold an overview of the many small steps involved or to sequence these over time. Problems in a number of domains—memory, visuospatial, motor—were probably also implicated in this , but poor organization was certainly present as well.

Those are the skill domains—attention, language, visuospatial, motor, executive, memory—and I check all these out to create a neurocognitive profile which helps me determine which skills are intact and which aren't, and this helps your physician or neurologist diagnose you more accurately and plan proper treatment.

Now let me make some observations. First, abilities such as those I have discussed above can be lost separately, a point I have made in different ways, but which I want to repeat here. You do not have to have memory problems to have language or visuospatial or motor problems. *Dementia* is a general term that implies neurocognitive losses in at least two domains, one of which must be memory, but you can suffer losses in other domains as well; when your losses are in those other domains but *not* in the domain of memory, you have a *cognitive disorder*. Also, Alzheimer's is a particular *kind* of dementia in which you must display significant inability to either learn new information or retrieve old information (visual or verbal) as well as deficits in at least one other domain, deficits due to a particular form of brain-cell pathology. In Vascular Dementia, it is blood vessel problems that lead to strokes and TIAs and other damage, and it is this damage that leads to losses in memory and other domains. There are also dementias due to other causes—Parkinson's disease, Huntington's disease, head injury, toxic exposure, infection, oxygen deprivation (e.g., near-drowning), and to various other medical or psychiatric disorders, and these all have characteristic presentations (usually). So *dementia* is just an umbrella term and *Alzheimer's* a specific type of dementia.

Second, cognitive deficits can interact. A poor visual memory is often made worse by visuospatial deficits, that is, if you cannot make a sense of a map or drawing, you are less likely to be able to structure it into memory, and poor internal maps make wandering about your neighborhood even more dangerous for you, and if you also have difficulty recalling where you live or speaking coherently, you may not be able to explain why or perhaps even *that* you are lost if someone tries to help you.

Third, after assessing roughly three thousand people of various ages, colors, religions, and socioeconomic situations, I have come to believe that we need to balance planning for old age with living in the present. I do not want to be alone and poor when I am old, so I worry about Social Security, savings, pensions, and all that, but I have also come to believe that the future is stubbornly unpredictable, that getting old at all is by no means guaranteed, and that an old age devoid of pleasant memories and the satisfaction of knowing that you lived out at least some of your dreams is not much to look forward to no matter how well you are being cared for. I meet too many old people who express regret, not for things they did, but for things they never got around to doing or were still saving up to do. So I save part of my income every pay period and cheerfully spend the rest on friends, theatre, books, my dogs, and other enthusiasms. If I learn tomorrow that I am dying, I will have few regrets (even though I will probably not be happy about the news).

Finally, after years of interest and training in meditation and in Eastern and Western religion and philosophies, and receiving my PhD from what was at the time considered a "New Age" school, the California Institute of Integral Studies in San Francisco, here I am working in a very medical area of psychology. What I want to say to you finally is this: If you are actively and consciously dealing with aging, disease or death in yourself or someone else, confronting the realities of these issues with or without professional healthcare training, you are performing the most spiritual work of all, whether you call it spiritual or not. It will reveal realities to you that no amount of reading or study can ever do. And if you do this work diligently and compassionately, you will reap enormous rewards. It will be more valuable to you than prayer, or sitting on a cushion with your eyes closed, or chanting (although such practices certainly have their own value). Moreover, your diligence will make this work more valuable to those you care for, right here and now, regardless of whether you or they believe in an afterlife or reincarnation. Such work makes us humane, not just human, and makes the world a better and warmer place. I highly recommend it.

References

Nuland, S. B. (1995). *How we die: Reflections on life's final chapter*. New York: Vintage.

5

The Aging Heart[3]

Doug Cort
Sandra Harner[4]

The Heart. It is so much more than a mere pump; so much more, that we often forget that it is also, fundamentally, a mere pump. In our language and our lives, the heart has come to stand for strength, goodness, compassion, love, and many other images and metaphors that connect us with the core of our being. Its absence, to be "heartless," signifies the most base, the most callous of human traits. Aging, too, has an important figurative aspect. It is so much more than adding time to our lives. It represents for many hopelessness, decline, and a loss of beauty and grace. For others, it represents acquisition of wisdom, balance in their lives, and even beauty. So, as we begin this chapter, we suspect that our essay titled *The Aging Heart* may bring up a multitude of images. And that would indeed be appropriate.

It is our belief that the aging heart is best understood by considering both physiology and metaphor as it describes human interactions. As we age, the chambers and vessels of the heart may thicken and harden. The pressure in the vessels often increases, and the efficiency of this most essential organ diminishes from long use. If that were the end of the story, this discussion would be over. This process of decline is predictable and yet can be significantly impacted both positively and negatively by our lifestyles. Healthful behaviors include concrete ones such as diet and exercise, but also behaviors that may seem more linked to the poetic or spiritual side of the heart. The way

---

[3] The following information is not intended as medical advice or to substitute for professional health care. Consult your physician for guidance in making lifestyle changes.

[4] The authors are grateful for the advice and support of C.T. Kappagoda, MD, PhD, Linda Aaron-Cort, and Michael Harner in the preparation of this chapter.

we feel toward ourselves and how we treat others may significantly affect the course of the aging heart. As we hope you will see, the poetry and physiology of the heart are inextricably entwined.

In normal aging, our likelihood of developing coronary disease increases. Our behavior can accelerate this process. We all know (though we may try to keep it out of our awareness) that normal aging involves physical decline. People who do not engage in health-promoting behaviors add insult to injury. It is normal that heart disease progresses.

Most of us do not think much about the heart during our younger years. It is just something that keeps on beating and does not seem to need much maintenance. Most of us have no idea how our hearts are faring. C.T. Kappagoda, Medical Director of the Preventive Cardiology Program at the University of California Davis Medical Center (UCDMC), has often said, "The first sign of heart problems is often a heart attack" (personal communication). It is for this reason he assembled a team to develop the Coronary Heart Disease Reversal Program (CHDRP). The team consists of individuals from multiple disciplines whose perspectives are integrated in a holistic effort to treat the heart patient. Over the years, the interdisciplinary team has reviewed and contributed to a growing body of research that clearly shows that behavior, feelings, and thoughts are powerful determinants for heart health.

The physical components of risk to heart health are well known. Less well known but, as you will see, equally important are the psychological and social elements. While physical and psychosocial factors affect all people, they may be especially relevant to those who are aging. If you attain the age of 70 and are a male you will have a 1 in 6 chance of having a heart attack or dying from one within 10 years (Expert Panel on Detection, Evaluation, and Treatment of High Blood Cholesterol in Adults, 2001). Women may have a lower likelihood, but the impact of individual risk factors is much greater. There is no doubt that getting older can be risky.

The adverse cardiac changes usually associated with normal aging may be accelerated through problems associated with poor resolution of the developmental issues of aging. Feelings of discouragement, hopelessness, social isolation, anger, and hostility increase susceptibility to heart disease. These may occur when the resolution of existential issues in aging is problematic. In other words, when a heartfelt connection with others is absent or problematic, it affects us physiologically. Two new and important pieces of research, the INTERHEART study and the *Normative Aging Study*, show the effects of psychosocial stress on the likelihood of heart attack most clearly (Yusuf et al., 2004; Kubzansky et al., 2006).

The INTERHEART Study had a huge international sample (approximately 30,000 people) and found that, no matter where in the world you live, the presence of psychosocial stress astronomically increases the likelihood of having a heart attack. If you have all the major physical risk factors (smoker, high blood pressure, high LDL or 'bad' cholesterol, and are obese), you are about 80 times more likely to have a heart attack than if you do not. But if you also have psychosocial stress (which the study defines as psychological stress at home and work, financial concerns, problematic locus of control [that is, your perceived ability to control your life circumstances], adverse life events, and depression), your risk jumps to almost *256* times greater.

From this study and many others, it is becoming clear that psychological variables independently add to or accelerate heart disease and diabetes. For example, the Metabolic Syndrome (MS) is now a well-established risk factor for heart disease. The Metabolic Syndrome is a collection of signs including abdominal obesity, high serum triglycerides, low serum HDL ('good' cholesterol), hypertension, and elevated blood sugar. If you have the Metabolic Syndrome, you are much more likely to develop coronary artery disease and 10% more likely to have a myocardial infarction (heart attack). However, if you have the MS and are hostile, you are 15% more likely to have a heart attack than if you have neither. Finally, in an example of interconnectedness, the MS is highly affected by lifestyle choices and stressors. This very same MS accounts for 50% of the attributable risk of developing Type 2 Diabetes (Todaro, 2005).

There are a number of psychological variables that accelerate heart disease (please see list on next page). As stated previously, the emotional challenges of aging may further increase the likelihood of problems occurring. Existential issues may lead to depression, anger or cynicism, isolation due to retirement, and financial concerns due to change in work status, income, and inflation. They can harden the heart both literally and figuratively.

While heart disease is the number one killer of both male and female Americans, the incidence is greatest in those 75 years of age and older. There is, however, some good news. We can do something about this situation by making behavioral and psychological changes necessary to stem the decline. By embracing these lifestyle changes, we can develop an integrated feedback system for reversing heart disease. Heart disease unfolds as we age and can be attended to and even reversed at any age by preventive measures and behaviors. Choosing to engage in heart-healthy practices early can maximize your chances for healthy aging.

Modifiable Physical Risk Factors for Coronary Heart Disease
- Smoking
- High Cholesterol
- High Blood Pressure
- Diabetes
- Overweight/Obesity
- Lack of Exercise or Physical Activity
- Diet High in Fat and Salt, Low in Fruits and Vegetables
- Alcohol Consumption Greater than 1 Drink Per Day for Women and 2 Per Day for Men

---

Modifiable Psychosocial Risk Factors for Coronary Heart Disease
- Psychological stress
- Financial concerns
- Helplessness to control important aspects of daily life
- Adverse life events
- Depression
- Anger and hostility
- High anxiety
- Little social support

Problems we create or do not address are in every way more difficult to deal with than problems we defer or prevent. It is harder to undo the effects of unhealthy behaviors than to prevent them. The time and energy it takes to heal is far greater and more difficult than to avoid sickness in the first place. This is not to say that we are completely the masters of our destiny, but we can have considerable influence on our present and future cardiac and general health.

The work done at The UCDMC Coronary Heart Disease Reversal Program in Sacramento, California may serve as a good example. The program's patients are men and women whose ages range from early thirties to the eighties. All have severe coronary atherosclerotic disease. Initially designed as a comprehensive two-year program, it combined state-of-the-art conventional medical treatment and rehabilitation with a healthy lifestyle program of information, practice, and monitoring. Nutrition, exercise, relaxation, meditation, psychological support groups, psycho-education, and individual psychotherapy as needed, are included regularly (Rutledge et al. 1999). Psychological testing is used to alert the staff and patients to factors that could potentiate or hamper their progress in the program (Cort et al. 1997, 1999). The extended length of the program itself supports patients as they develop new habits of a heart-healthy lifestyle, including psychologically "softening" the heart. While the program has altered its scope, the benefits continue.

Here is some of what Kappagoda et al. (2006) found during our work with these patients. *Of the people who completed the program by doing 60 percent or more of its requirements, less than 3 percent had another cardiac event within 10 years. Those who failed to complete the program had a re-event rate of more than 20 percent and those who never did the program were in the 30 percent or higher range. The people who completed the program had less depression, anxiety, and anger, as well as fewer somatic concerns.* This is important because both anxiety and depression are critical psychological factors that place a person at risk for developing heart disease. Anxiety and depression also normally accompany the major trauma of heart disease, heart attack, and coronary bypass surgery.

Life Span Development

Psychological development across the life span is relevant to avoiding heart disease. Erik Erikson presented a model of dynamic biopsychosocial developmental stages throughout one's lifespan (Erikson, 1950, 1986), including middle and old age, the very periods when heart disease is most likely to become evident. His model envisioned three explicit aspects: the physical body, the psychological processes, and the social-cultural context. Each has its own set of knowledge and research methods, yet they profoundly impact one another. He proposed that throughout life we face a sequence of psychosocial crises or focal tensions. When each crisis is met successfully enough, there emerges a strength that prepares us for the next stage of development.

In middle adulthood, the core crisis, "Generativity vs. Stagnation," focuses on the matter of caring for the next generation. Generativity may be viewed literally, as in parenting, or viewed metaphorically, such as in mentoring, teaching, or creating products and ideas of value for ensuing generations. The issue is one of a genuine concern for them and their future. The polar opposite of generativity, which Erickson termed stagnation, is reflected in a lack of interest, or frank rejection of, those who are of a younger generation. Failure to adequately meet the challenge of generativity leaves the individual inadequately prepared for the next stage of development.

Erikson's last stage of adult psychosocial development, old age, involves the core conflict of "Integrity versus Despair" (Erikson, 1950, 1986). From a satisfactory resolution of this polarity comes wisdom, which Erikson described as "the detached concern with life in the face of death itself" (Erikson, 1982). Integrity speaks to a consolidation and acceptance of life experience with equanimity, leading to wisdom, while despair leads to disdain for self and others in the face of physical, psychological, and social decline.

If resolution of these developmental challenges is so unbalanced in favor of either of the antithetical elements of the core conflicts that the other is atrophied, maladaptation may result. However, it is important to note that in Erikson's model the choice is not an "either-or" situation. Both aspects are necessary, but the positive must outweigh the negative in order for the person to be able to meet the usual and inevitable challenges of life. One of these challenges is attending to declining health as we age. How we meet such developmental crises throughout our lives impacts how we respond to the demands of illness, compliance with treatment, and our changed social engagement.

Advancing age can become a time of discovery of those developmental aspects that one has not yet successfully negotiated in the context of present realities. It is also a time to resolve further the developmental stages Erikson proposed and to find unknown resources within.

To develop a lifestyle that decreases the likelihood of heart disease and to promote a lifestyle that is cardio-protective requires a willingness to change one's perspective. Facing some hard truths, patients must identify and practice new behaviors that are active ingredients in both the prevention and reversal of heart disease. Harder yet, they need to make fundamental lifestyle changes and challenge unhealthy habits once they are established and disease has set in. This requires discipline and motivation.

What elements may be active ingredients in both prevention and reversal of heart disease? The process of altering our perspective requires acceptance of the following truths. First, we are biological beings; second, life is terminal; and third, we can make choices. Finally, the fourth truth is that we live in a social context that constantly exerts pressures, both positive and negative.

We have intentionality and, therefore, our decisions and behaviors can be goal-directed. But in the end, for all our choosing, motivations, intentions, and discipline, we are limited in what we can control. In the face of unknowns, a fundamental commitment to a way of life with full awareness is necessary to make lifestyle choices and changes effectively. To confront these realities skillfully in the moment is a challenge, which impacts our physical, emotional, and philosophical concepts of "heart."

A broad view of ourselves is required to maximize our health and potential. We must address physical considerations, but also must consider the psychological context. We are affected by existential issues, which, like cholesterol levels or other physical markers, we ignore at our peril. This existential and humanistic perspective of mature adult development is reflected in the works of psychotherapists such as Viktor Frankl, James F. T. Bugental, Rollo May, and Abraham Maslow. They support a view of the adult potential that also addresses emotional challenges and health issues, particularly aging and its accompanying health problems, as well as maximizing each individual's creative potential and personal meaning (see especially Bugental, 1981 & 1999).

Contemporary psychological theory has increasingly focused on health. This perspective is called positive psychology and its exponents include Martin Seligman, B.L. Fredrickson, Mihalyi Csikszentmihalyi, and others. While personal decline is inevitable, truly difficult times may be postponed. Indeed, we now strongly suspect that surviving and thriving have at least as much to do with the presence of positive attitudes and variables as with the absence of negative ones (Fredrickson, 2001). Positive psychology is the scientific study of ordinary human strengths and virtues, finding out what works, what is right, and what is improving. Normal functioning cannot be accounted for by just looking through negative or problem-focused frames of reference (Sheldon & King, 2001). Positive emotions, such as joy, optimism, interest, gratitude, contentment, and love, may all serve as markers of optimal well-being and are well worth cultivating (Fredrickson, 2001). The field of positive psychology looks at, among other things, capacity for love and vocation, courage, interpersonal skill, aesthetic sensibility, perseverance, forgiveness, and wisdom (Seligman & Csikszentmihalyi, 2000).

Indeed, positive feelings and behaviors may be associated with an open heart, both literally and figuratively. Fredrickson (2001) talks about how specific emotions may lead to specific tendencies of action. For example, fear leads to wanting to escape, and anger to an urge to attack. Positive emotions such as acceptance and love may well translate into behavior geared to approach, rather than avoid, and lead to more frequent and satisfying social interactions and support. It is well established that the degree of social support correlates with development of, and recovery from, heart disease (e.g., Gomer et al., 1993). Developing positive emotions may help mitigate the effects of stress and improve coping (Folkman, 1997). Studies have shown that people who experience positive emotions during bereavement are more likely to develop long-term plans and goals (Stein, Folkman, Trabasso & Richards, 1997).

Optimism and other positive feelings have an effect on attractiveness, approach behaviors, and motivation to engage in healthy activities. Conversely, high levels of stress and negative emotions may well lead to illness because of supporting behaviors such as eating unhealthy food, abusing alcohol and drugs, and poor sleep, all relevant to heart disease and other lifestyle diseases.

Recent research reveals that in addition to the release of corticosteroids (stress hormones), stress impacts heart health through the immune system by setting off an inflammatory response most likely through increased interleukin 6 (IL-6) (Kiecolt-Glaser, et al., 2003). The chronic presence of an increased level of this proinflammotory protein can thus lead to chronic inflammation and to heart disease, as well as to other age-related disorders such as arthritis, osteoporosis, and Type II diabetes. Furthermore, aging itself, as well as depressive symptoms and clinical depression, can also activate an inflammatory response through the IL-6 pathway. Beyond stress, other behaviors that increase the amount of IL-6 are smoking, a high-fat diet, poor sleep, and inadequate exercise.

Social aspects of aging and illness take on very personal meanings when we or someone close to us gets sick. As part of the lived experience, these meanings may be expressed differently by each of us. The underlying challenge of change is nearly inevitable; change not only for the patient, but also for the patient's nearest and dearest. Family, caregivers, friends, work, and recreation can all be dramatically affected. Nor is there a linear or direct relation of cause and effect. A whole system can be thrown into chaos by one person's serious, debilitating illness. With each subtle or not-so-subtle change comes the opportunity to face the realities of life in a way that may have otherwise escaped serious notice. Thus, heart health requires preventing heart disease where we can *and* coping with the illness we are unable to avoid. It may also suggest openness to the important and potentially life-affirming and enhancing lessons that illness may provide.

Some of the floundering questions of youth are stilled in the context of illness, aging, and imminent death. Existential issues that were in the background earlier take on new meaning in the context of the lived present. In first brushes with a physical crisis, the priority is for meeting the needs of the emergency. Against this plays a looming recognition of mortality, with all the accompanying pressures that awareness of it brings.

Aging and its attendant challenges can be an invitation to a personal future with greater understanding – and an opportunity to answer nagging questions about meaning in our lives based on our own direct experiences. The reality is that for most of us, the "learning experiences" of aging and illness must wait to be absorbed as we deal with the immediate and unfolding events, whether as the person directly affected or as close companions. The required responses are usually multi-faceted, sometimes sequential and, more often, simultaneous. To find so much of life changed suddenly, and in many ways, can knock us out of our daily trance and into a foreign landscape, internally and externally.

Lives can change unimaginably. Coping with the unknown, the unforeseen, becomes the order of the day. We are both player and witness in the drama. Our physical resources and our abilities to recover in a timely fashion may be diminished. The evidence of the interdependence of the physical and emotional aspects of being demands fresh appraisals of our limitations and potentialities.

The role of the individual within a system comes into sharp focus as the impact of illness makes its way through relationships. No longer can we maintain long-held illusions of ourselves as independent. We find that however independent we may have been as individuals, we are ultimately part of a larger network. And that network is affected by illness or injury to one of its own. The responses of those within the social fabric may vary considerably depending on how and where its members are meeting their own developmental challenges. One may be met with unprecedented kindness from some. Some may become fearful, others may become angry and flee in righteous indignation and blame, and others may rally to support within their own limits and understandings. Compassion and social skills can meet within the context of deeper understanding. Keeping hope alive may be the single most important ability in coping with the bid to meet the new moment.

The Good News

All this news and the seemingly hard solutions may seem discouraging, with change at the core of stress. But change is also at the core of any solution. One's willingness to change can make a big difference in outcome. In the UCDMC Heart Disease Reversal Program model, those who completed a regimen that aimed at changing problematic lifestyle patterns effectively avoided having another serious cardiac event. As indicated earlier, those who started the program but did not finish it fared better than individuals who never tried, yet they still had a 20-percent greater chance of an event than those who completed the program. The results indicate that successful behavioral changes make big differences and show that any move in the right direction is better than nothing.

Risk factors can be measured and modified. They are not isolated from each other, but part of a combination of behaviors. A coordinated effort of a few actions will have a cascading effect on a number of these systems and risks. For example, a heart-healthy diet can contribute to weight loss, and with it, a loss of excess fat, which, in turn, may reduce blood cholesterol levels. As the function of blood vessels improves, blood pressure may decrease and diabetes become better controlled, together reducing the risk of heart disease *and* even reversing its progress. Exercise can increase the level of HDL (*the 'good' cholesterol*), contribute further to weight loss, lower blood pressure, and reduce stress. Smoking cessation leads to, among other things, increased beneficial HDL and healthier blood vessels. Introducing stress reduction experiences such as meditation, relaxation, and yoga can lower high blood pressure, increase coping ability, physically and emotionally, and address the psychological stresses we have discussed.

These are important choices you can make. They are under your control and can have far-reaching positive effects on your health. Work with your health care providers to develop a custom-made plan specific for you – and stick to it! It may include exercise, diet, medication, and other components. Keeping records of your behaviors and progress, and regularly reviewing them with your health care professional, can help keep you on track in meeting your goals.

There are additional ways of maximizing your success. For instance, prioritize your proposed changes. Start with the one most important to you. Slowly add other changes. Celebrate as you meet each goal. Seek support. It may be found among those close to you, as well as through other options, such as consulting a clinical or health psychologist or other mental health care provider specializing in this field. Such consultations may help you clarify to yourself the meaning of the changes, and provide motivation and support as you set about to meet the tasks you have planned.

Concluding Thoughts

The connection between emotion and health has been observed and even emphasized for thousands of years. The National Library of Medicine notes

> ...Hippocrates (ca. 460 B.C. 370 B.C.) and his followers combined naturalistic craft knowledge with ancient science and philosophy to produce the first systematic explanations of the behavior of the human body in health and illness. ... They made the first attempts to understand emotions as mental phenomena which had surprising and complex connections to physiological order and pathological disorder. (National Library of Medicine, n.d.)

Aging, if not approached mindfully, may lead to despair, sadness, loneliness, and a resulting increased risk of heart disease. But if we are able to be more emotionally positive, the opposite can occur. This outcome works through several pathways. The direct route is probably the least understood. We do know that chronic stress and negative emotions lead to the release of stress hormones that decrease immune functioning while increasing blood pressure, cholesterol levels, and even weight. We have discussed research showing that negative feelings and behaviors, such as anger, depression, and social isolation, are risk factors for heart disease. We are fortunate to live in a time where health-related science is beginning to focus on strength and health instead of just infirmity and disease.

Some risk factors cannot be changed, such as age, gender, and genetic makeup. Therefore, it is important to focus on the ones you *can* change because the cumulative and synergistic effect of risk factors is most harmful to our hearts. The psychosocial aspects are major amplifiers of the disease process, but they can be modulated. Make lifestyle changes that have a real positive impact on your longevity and quality of life. These can delay, and potentially minimize, disability as you age. You can make a difference in your own health and aging.

As you have seen, heart disease and health are inextricably tied with psychological health and habits. Our acquired behaviors and habits are shaped early on by such things as our family, culture, education and socio-economic status. We practice them uncritically so they become essentially out of our daily awareness. Psychologists may refer to them as over-learned behaviors similar to, for example, riding a bike. Heart disease, too, progresses outside our awareness – until something critical "wakes us up." This wake-up call can be a painful gift. If you do experience this, remember: Old dogs can indeed learn new tricks. Problematic behaviors can be unlearned and we can acquire new healthier ones. Adult development is in many ways as dynamic and important as in youth. Indeed, the great news is that the aging process may bring an improved quality of life.

There are some very specific things you may do to affect this, regardless of your known cardiac status. George Vaillant and his colleagues tracked a number of people to identify what contributed to positive aging (see Vaillant, 2003). Their results suggest that social and emotional maturation may be associated with aging and thus confer an improved outlook and decreased stress. The emotional maturation associated with aging is really about the development of increasingly adaptive coping mechanisms. We all know how aging seldom leads to faster reflexes or visual acuity. However, "increased strength" may come from being better able to cope with what we are given. In doing so, we decrease the impact of many of the variables that are so harmful to us, such as anger, depression and social isolation.

We hope this chapter serves as a gentle alarm clock, awakening you to the potential of a new day with your heart strong, and filled with love, support and hope.

References

Bugental, J.F.T. (1991). *The search for authenticity: An existential-analytic approach to psychotherapy* (Enlarged edition). New York: Irvington.

Bugental, J. F. T. (1999). *Psychotherapy isn't what you think: Bringing the psychotherapeutic engagement into the living moment*. Phoenix: Zeig, Tucker.

Cort, D., Harner, S., Kappagoda, T., Neuhaus, E., & Rutledge, J. (1997). Program decreases depression, anxiety, somatic concerns and cardiovascular events. *Proceedings of the Society of Behavioral Medicine, Annals of Behavioral Medicine, 19*, S14 (Supplement).

Cort, D., Harner, S., Roman, M., Morrison, T, & Kappagoda, T. (1999). MMPI changes in patients attending the Coronary Heart Disease Reversal Program (CHDRP) at the University of California, Davis

Medical Center (UCDMC). *Proceedings of the Society of Behavioral Medicine, Annals of Behavioral Medicine, 21,*S039 *(Supplement).*

Erikson, E. (1965). *Childhood and society.* New York: Norton. (Original work published in 1950)

Erikson, E. (1982). *The life cycle completed.* New York: Norton.

Erikson, E., Erikson, J., & Kivnick, H. (1986). *Vital involvement in old age.* New York: Norton.

Expert Panel on Detection, Evaluation, and Treatment of High Blood Cholesterol in Adults. (2001). Executive summary of third report of the National Cholesterol Education Program (NCEP) Expert Panel on Detection, Evaluation, and Treatment of High Blood Cholesterol in Adults (Adult Treatment III), *JAMA, 285,* 2486-2497.

Folkman, S. (1997). Positive psychological states and coping with severe stress. *Social Science Medicine, 45,* 1207-1221.

Fredrickson, B. L. (2001). The role of positive emotions in positive psychology. *American Psychologist, 56,* 218-226.

Kappagoda, C.T., May, A., Cort, D. A., Paumer, L., Lucas, D., Burns, J., & Amsterdam, E. (2006) Cardiac Event Rate in the Lifestyle Modification Program for Patients with Chronic Coronary Artery Disease. *Clinical Cardiology, 29,* 317-321.

Kiecolt-Glaser, J.K., Preacher, K.J., MacCallum, R.C., Atkinson, C., Malarkey, W.B., & Glaser, R. (2003). Chronic stress and age-related increases in the Proinflammatory cytokine IL-6. *Proceedings of the National Academy of Sciences USA, 100,* 9090-9095.

Kubzansky L.D., Cole S.R., Kawachi I., Vokonas P., & Sparrow, D. (2006). Shared and unique contributions of anger, anxiety, and depression to coronary heart disease: a prospective study in the normative aging study. *Annals of Behavioral Medicine, 31,* 21-29.

National Library of Medicine. History of Medicine Division. (n.d.). Emotions and Disease. *The balance of passions.* Retrieved November 21, 2008, from http://www.nlm.nih.gov/hmd/emotions.html

Orth-Gomer, K., Rosengren, A., & Wilhelmsen, L. (1993). Lack of social support and incidence of coronary heart disease in middle-aged Swedish men. *Psychosomatic Medicine,* Jan-Feb, *55* (1): 37-4.

Rutledge, J.D., Hyson, D.A., Garduno, D., Cort, D.A., Paumer, L., & Kappagoda, C.T. (1999). Lifestyle modification program in management of patients with coronary artery disease: the clinical experience in a tertiary care hospital. *Journal of Cardiopulmonary Rehabilitation, 19*(4), 226-343.

Salovey, P., Rothman, A., Detweiler, J., & Steward, W. (2000). Emotional states and physical health. *American Psychologist, 55,* 110-121.

Seligman, M. E. & Csikszentmihalyi, M. (2000). Positive psychology, An introduction. *American Psychologist, 55,* 5-14.

Sheldon, K. M. & King, L. (2001). Why positive psychology is necessary. *American Psychologist, 56,* 216-217.

Stein, N. L., Folkman, S., Trabasso, T., & Richards, T. A. (1997). Appraisal and goal processes as predictors of psychological well-being in bereaved caregivers. *Journal of Personality and Social Psychology, 72,* 872-884.

Todaro, J.F., Con, A., Niaura, R., Spiro, A. 3rd, Ward, K.D., & Roytberg, A. (2005). Combined effect of the metabolic syndrome and hostility on the incidence of myocardial infarction (the Normative Aging Study). *American Journal of Cardiology, 96*(2), 221-226.

Vaillant, G. (2003). *Aging well.* Boston: Little Brown and Co.

Yusuf, S., Hawken, S., Ounpuu, S., Dans, T., Avezum, A., Lanas, F., et al. (2004). Effect of potentially modifiable risk factors associated with myocardial infarction in 52 countries (the INTERHEART study): case-control study. *Lancet, 364*(9438), 937-952.

6

Aging:
Facing the Inevitable Facts of Life

Regina Reilly

Writing about growing old has been more challenging for me than I first imagined. Calling it aging does not make it any easier. I would not be even thinking about it if I were not growing older. You might say I am less and less able to stay in denial about the facts of life.

I did not think about it much before I began to notice certain physical and psychological changes. These changes brought up deep questions that, as a younger person, I was only intellectually interested in. Now, however, they have an immediacy that gives them a seat in the front row of my mind. Yes, and they go beyond my mind as I ponder the very nature of what I am, and who I am, and what a human life is for anyway.

How does one talk about aging? Because I want to pass on some wisdom and not just fill up space with words, I am going to tell you stories about the aging processes people dear to me experienced.. When you come right down to it, growing old is what happens to all creatures that are born, if they live long enough; that means that each experience of aging is unique and deserves a voice. If all of us who are aging speak of it, a rich legacy of collective wisdom will be passed on to future human generations.

Mother's Wisdom

My mother, after raising seven souls to adulthood, with my father, and living with my father and us and our dog in a small house, finally found herself living alone in a house of her own. My father had died; all of us had married and moved into homes of our own. You might think that having a home to herself would be a lovely experience for her, one she earned with all the years of cooking and doing for others. On the contrary, living alone was difficult for her. It seemed unnatural; "too quiet," she would say. My sister, Kate, her seventh child, saw that she was lonely. So she went to the animal shelter and got her a dog, Molly.

Molly came to live with Mom at precisely the right time in their lives. Neither was young; neither had any particular reason for living, nothing that demanded they take care of anything. Life was just the living of it day by day. They were seldom apart once they met each other. For instance, they would sit together on the couch in front of the television. Mom would make tea and put the cup and pot on a TV table (furniture out of the 50's!) and she and Molly would watch television and have tea. Naturally, Molly did not drink tea. Mom did. Now the cookies—that was the sharing part: "one cookie for you, one for me" is how they passed many hours. Her adult children clucked and rolled our eyes! But we knew in our hearts that our mother, who wanted each of us to have our own lives without having to care for her in any special way, really needed the warmth and the aliveness and the affection of Molly.

People who are growing old need the companionship and contact and warm feeling that comes from being with familiar people and animals. Living creatures make all the difference. They may not have the energy to do all the activity that they once did. Nonetheless, they need to be *with* others in daily, active ways.

One day in the fall, which was her favorite time of year, my mother was watering a plant that she had hung from the ceiling in the kitchen. The kitchen was at the back of the house facing out on the back yard. Toting the watering can, she climbed up the steps of the ladder, watered the plant, and on the way down, she missed her step and fell hard onto the kitchen floor. She could not move. She was near the door from the kitchen out to the garage, but the garage door was closed.

There she sat for some time, because every time she moved, there was pain and she knew she had broken something. At first, she called out for help, but soon tired of that. People in her neighborhood did not go out walking much and she knew that it was unlikely that anyone would hear her. She could not get to the phone, so she said a prayer, and waited.

I have no idea how long she lay there, but she tells the story that she could hear the dog next door barking on and off. When Molly was alive, she would take her for a walk and that dog would run along the fence around the yard and play with Molly as they went. More and more, the dog barked and barked until finally the woman who owned her came out and told her to quiet down. Mom called out for help and continued yelling as loud as she could until the woman heard her.

"Where are you?" the woman asked.

"I'm in the kitchen. The garage door is unlocked. If you can raise it up, you can get in here through the garage. I can't get up. I fell down!" said my mother trying to prepare her for what she was about to find.

The woman yelled through the garage door, "I'll go get my husband. I'll be right back!"

The dog had quit barking. It was very quiet now as my mother lay on the floor waiting to be rescued. "In the silence," she said, "I felt the blessing of that dog; I realized that I am not alone, and I knew I'd be all right."

Her friends and neighbors spoke of it as a terrible thing that happened to her, but my mother managed the surgery, the hip replacement, and the months of physical therapy with grace and humor. For the most part, that is. There were days when her mood would be contentious. A foul mood would come over her for a while and she would sit in bed with no desire to get going. We worried, and we let her be. We stayed around, but we did not draw her out. She obviously needed that time to stew or digest or reconstitute her inner life in her own way.

Over the years, more and more the focus of her attention turned from her activity in the church and with her grandchildren to her health. She was fortunate in that she was very sensible and resilient. When she found out that she was diabetic, she took insulin and changed her diet. Eventually, she managed to get off the insulin and with exercise and eating "according to the rules" as she would say, managed her diabetes There were times she would cheat: She and her children would go out to dinner and she would have a good old time. "I'll pay tomorrow, but it's worth the price," she'd say.

There were two hip replacements. There was the operation on her eyes for cataracts, which was such a success as it enabled her to read again without glasses. Then there was the cleaning out of her carotid arteries. She had been feeling so fatigued. After the cleaning, her energy was great and she was up and active again. The last big diagnosis, and the one that she could not conquer, was congestive heart failure.

The quantity and variety of medications that she had to organize and ingest was staggering to me. They changed over the years as she aged and went through the above-mentioned journeys with her body needing care and treatment. My sister, Carol, the third child, is a nurse and she was my mother's advocate in dealing with doctors and hospitals. Now my mother, strong as she was, was born and lived at a time when doctors and all people in authority positions were to be followed because they knew best. It is a mystery to me how as someone intelligent and willful as she could be would be so willing to surrender her own judgment and intuitive knowing to the doctor or the authority of another. So my sister, Carol, would get the information from the doctor or the physician's assistant or nurse, size up the situation, request the tests or evaluations which my mother would never have asked for, and get as complete a picture as possible. This would take time, of course.

Then she would sit down with my mother (usually one or more of us would be there, too) and present her with the information, bit by bit, until all the pieces of the picture were clear to her. This, too, would take place over several visits when the situation was complex. These conversations required mother to participate in her own health care. Her participation ensured that she was making choices rather than being treated as if she were a child or incompetent. She was openly appreciative of that respect.

At one point, it seemed clear to Carol and to us that her doctor was not providing satisfactory care. He kept adding medications and she was not feeling better. One medication was interfering with another, we found out, and in general her body was not able to manage what was being ingested. In fact, we found there was toxicity arising from the medications themselves. She was "fuzzy" in her head, she would say, and could not make sense out of this. But she was reluctant to get another doctor because she did not want to hurt his feelings. She could be amazingly stubborn about something like this even when it meant that her health would suffer.

My sister had a conversation with the nurse in the clinic and found out that this doctor was planning to retire in two years so that he was not taking on any new patients. Carol was able to bring that information to Mom in a way that let her feel free to get another doctor. This new doctor, indeed, took her off all medication and conducted tests, and prescribed medications that were needed. She still took a lot of pills, from my point of view, but she knew what she was taking, and what each one was for, and she was clear that she was a participant in the process. But, of course, the doctor was still the authority who knew best for her! I had to accept that this is the way she was.

Being around my mother and father and their friends as they were growing old did nothing to wake me up to the facts or the vicissitudes of aging. It is sobering to realize that for many years of my life I harbored a denial that I would lose the energy and capacities that I had grown accustomed to experiencing and felt entitled to as my life. "Sobering" is the word that describes my dawning realization that aging is a biological happening and it is happening to me. Furthermore, it has nothing whatsoever to do with whether I want it or not. It started to come over me like tiny invisible drops of water in a mist slowly sinking into my skin and bones, and yes, into my consciousness. It gradually sinks in and it affects everything. My energy changed from high to low in unpredictable cycles; my health suddenly became an issue; my schedule was riddled with doctor's appointments because I have to have regular tests: blood tests, diabetes test, bone density tests, blood pressure tests, and so on. In addition, dental health now needed more attention. Supplements begin to usurp a large proportion of my income! How could this be happening to me? I secretly rage in part of myself. How disappointing that I am an ordinary human being, simply aging. Resist as I might, I do not lose my practical nature: I do take care of business.

As I write about this, I realize that coping with my aging process is more daunting than getting through graduate school was for me. In order to make sense of what was going on in my body, I decided to treat it like a research project. I love to learn and the research project reframed it so I could relate to it with a more positive attitude.

As I discovered the biological data available in articles about aging or more fondly put, becoming an elder, memories of my father came back to me. Images of him in his late 60's sitting in his Lazy-Boy recliner staring at Hoss Cartwright on his horse in *Bonanza* are still vivid. A frown on his face, his left hand cupped around his ear, he strained to hear.

Lessons from My Father

At 70, he railed against his failing body. He was a farmer and was used to being strong and working hard physically. He had held many jobs in his life. He had been a deputy sheriff and in his final job, he was the warden of the county jail. He, according to an article in the newspaper, did a fine job running that jail. Another surprise! I would never have imagined that he could administer anything. My mother did that. Dad was an outdoors man and he was very seldom sick. We all looked askance at this aging father and pretended not to notice that he was losing ground. He didn't talk about it at all.

One day as he was hoeing tomatoes or maybe it was the corn, he had a "spell," which is our codeword for something bad happening, which told us he was sick. He was diagnosed with late onset diabetes.

He always called the doctor "they" so he told us, before they want me to give myself an injection of insulin every day. He was incredulous. That was so impossible as far as he was concerned, it was not even funny.

But that was not the worst of it. They told him he had to stop drinking beer. That was a blow he took like a personal insult. I had no idea that he would react so vehemently. But as I sorted it out from his point of view, it made perfect sense. When you try to understand someone who is aging, you have to get into their skin and look out and feel it from their point of view. From his point of view, this was a terrible loss.

Of course, he became depressed. Not only was he having to take in all this medicine that he, as a man of the earth and natural foods did not like one little bit, but also he was told he had to stop drinking beer, actually, all alcohol. That was a bitter pill because my father's social life consisted of life at the pub, a small bar where he could hang out with his cronies and shoot darts, play euchre (cards), tell stories, and of course, drink a beer or two. My father must have felt that to give up beer and the fun and friends that went along with it was to die in some way, because although he pretended to follow instructions, he actually never stopped drinking beer. Additionally, the side effects from the medications cause him to feel sick most of the time.

My mother was tracking his pills each day, and they disappeared, but I think she chose not to push it or him. I thought he had given up on life, but after his funeral, when we were telling the stories about when he started to "go downhill," I learned that he had his own ideas about what made his life worth living. Now I see that it is more compassionate to respect that. Possibly, he had been depressed for many years of his life and was too busy raising plants, animals, and children to notice it. The beer and the friends may have lightened the load, the responsibility that he carried as the father of the family. I can find room in my heart not to judge harshly. On the other hand, the physical body was, no doubt, tired; he had been working hard since a boy of nine years, when his dad would get him up at four a.m. to harness up the horses and go to market to sell the produce. His brain, his liver, and his kidneys had been strong, but when the pancreas stopped producing the insulin he needed, that caused a quantum leap in his aging.

Another factor that influenced his aging was that, in my view, he was stubborn and rigid in his thinking. I can see that I am like him in this way at times. It was as if he was entitled to be healthy forever or at least as long as he lived. He was incensed that this should happen to him. He would say really silly things like, "getting old is an awful thing!

Don't ever get old," shaking his head. He was deeply identified with a strong, healthy, energetic body. He could not roll with this punch as my mother could. He resisted every inch of the way, and he died a hard death. I hope he's resting peacefully now.

He used to tell me I was thick. He would say, "Well kid, there's no sense in being Irish if you can't be thick!" He had a way of teasing and laughing, but it sure had a sting to it. That same character trait made it really hard to comfort him as he aged. He had a hard time taking in our love. We loved him and craved to take his wrinkled face in our hands and say, "Don't you know how precious you are to us?" Sadly, that never happened.

He just did not like slowing down and feeling limits, and he was set against it in a willful way. He had to have surgery to remove his prostate. He got a staph infection while in the hospital and the doctor wanted him to have around-the-clock nursing so he was moved to a nursing home when it was time to leave the hospital.

He was miserable. He was fighting mad. His condition deteriorated although the foot, where the staph infection had flared up, appeared to heal. The infection went inside and the doctor decided to amputate his leg above the knee. I saw him once before the surgery. He was so sick! It was shocking to see this father of mine who was sick maybe once or twice in his life weak and suffering. I still feel the horror and the sadness of it when I contemplate that time of his life. You might have guessed that he did not come out of that surgery. "Renal failure" said the report. Refusal to live without his leg is what I say. I am sad for him, and I do not blame him a bit for not hanging around.

Sometimes I think of W.H. Auden's poem to his father: "Do not go gentle into that good night." On the contrary, I wish my father could have relaxed and faced his dying with some sense of the love that surrounded him, some sense that life offers death as it does birth, and that he hadn't failed by getting sick and getting old. I wish he could have rolled with the punches, as she would say and accepted his dying as the natural next movement of his soul in his life.

Now that I have felt the loss of both mother and father, it seems clear to me that older people often are afraid of feeling many of their feelings and wind up becoming depressed. And the adult children of older folks are afraid of depression, too. That is part of what makes it difficult to let yourself know you are aging: there is so much you do not want to feel or experience. The death of friends and colleagues, and especially siblings, looms as you age. Coming to accept that life here on earth and our physical bodies are temporary is a big task. If we do it, we have matured; if we do not, we suffer because we resist the movement of our soul in its journey in life.

Getting old requires time. Of course, you say. But, I mean time to sit down and ponder what life really is. Experience is not just going places and doing things. Experience is feeling the sensations in your body even when they are aches and pains. Those make it even more delicious when you find yourself feeling sexy, lively, or free of pain. Somehow the focus and value as I age move from doing or being active to experiencing the aliveness I feel in myself. Standing still and listening to the birds can make me aware of the oneness of everything and I know I am blessed.

I live alone in a wonderful home. What is it like to age and live alone? I am now contemplating that each day of my life. I know I do not want to become dependent on somebody, lose my mobility, my freedom to go where I want, when I want. I do not want to lose the ability to make my own choices and to have to follow orders from somebody else even if they are for my own good. I do not want to lose the capacity to read, hear music, handle my horse, pull weeds out of my flower beds, have a beer with a friend, eat a meal, climb a ladder and not fall down, swim, walk a steep trail, lift a 20-pound bag of cat food, or drive a car. All these are markers of life to me. I recognize that I will lose at least some of them. Facing that, I turn my attention more and more inward. I look inside and feel. I find life is vibrant in my inner world. Not in my mind, mentally, like in fantasy or imagination, but in my soul where I connect with life on a deep level.

I often reflect on the words of Elizabeth Kubler-Ross (1986) who saw aging and dying as the final phase of growth in earthly life. I, on the other hand, have believed getting old was a lessening of life experience, a diminishment of sorts, and so have not wanted to face that it would one day come upon me. Much to my surprise I am discovering that life is no less vital; in fact, that my spirit is younger, wilder and freer than ever before. Yes, I have discovered that life is full of surprises—even as you become elderly.

The thing about my mother's situation that was very different from mine was that in her old age, she was the mother of seven adults, the grandmother of 24 children of various ages, and several great-grandchildren. Some of these young people were able to drive a car, and loved to come and take her out for an adventure. As you see, she had people around her who were in touch on a continual basis, both for fun times and when she needed to be taken to the doctor, or some such thing more serious.

My life is quite different: I live alone in a rural area, up on a mountain. Not quite alone—I have a horse and two cats, but they don't drive and would be of no help if I needed to get to a hospital. I often wonder what will happen to me if I break a hip or have a stroke. In many ways I am still young. But my friends do evoke the reality of aging as they talk about their concerns for themselves and for me. Of course, this conversation shows you I am thinking about it; I even have bought long-term care insurance.

I love my home and I am still working, although I am over the age when it is customary to retire. I daydream with my women friends about pooling our money and buying a big Victorian home in town, one with a big kitchen, many bathrooms, and a wrap-around porch where we could all rock in our favorite chairs and play cards, or knit, and tell stories about the absurd things, the wonderful and terrifying things that have happened to us in our lives. I guess that would feel like the home I grew up in. There was always someone around.

I really like living alone, but it does concern me as I grow older. As long as my health holds, I can manage my few acres and keep my head above water. But there probably will come a time when, like my mother, I will have to bite the bullet and change my living situation. However, my intention is to be creative about it, not wait "till the time is upon me" and I have no choice. I will live each day in the wonder of not knowing how I will do it. Then maybe in ten years I'll look back and say, "Well, look at that! I've been coping with aging for all these years and I didn't know how to do it."

As I am sure you can see better than I, I am like my father in ways and like my mother in ways. So I will see if I can find a way to be old and have my community of friends around me rather than strangers in an assisted living home. Or perhaps I will manage to live alone until one day I will simply sit down in one of my rocking chairs near my pond under the old oak tree, and peacefully fall asleep, having looked happily for the last time at the golden orange sunset reflected in the still water.

References

Kubler-Ross, E. (1986). *Death: The final stage of growth*. New York: Touchstone.

Part 3

Gifts for the Journey:
Walking the Talk

7

What Am I Doing Here: A Psychologist's Reflections on Providing Care to Nursing Home Residents

Christopher S. M. Grimes

Do you ever ask yourself, "What am I doing here?" During my two years working part-time providing psychological assessment and treatment to nursing home residents, I asked myself this question quite a bit. Geriatric psychology was not a specialty with which I had planned to get involved. Initially, I took the position to supplement the private practice caseload I was still working to build. At the time, I had just completed my post-doctoral residency and was eager to begin earning a living, but I found building a private practice caseload large enough to provide sufficient income was not an overnight thing. So, when approached by Behavioral Health Partners regarding a position providing psychological services to nursing home facilities, I decided to give it a try.

I write this chapter not as an expert in geriatric psychology, but to share my experience, hopefully with some benefit for others. My graduate training was focused on adult clinical psychology, with not much emphasis on the geriatric age group. Practically all of my clinical experience to this point had been with individuals age 60 or younger. When I went to interview with Margaret Barger, the Vice President of BHP, I had this thought in the back of my head, "What am I doing here?" The idea of working in a nursing facility had not entered my mind until I heard about the job opening with BHP. Nonetheless, I received the job, and a few weeks later I was being introduced to nursing home administrators and staff in the facilities I would be serving. Again during those first days and weeks on the job, in the back of my mind was that question: "What am I doing here?" Through this chapter of reflection, I hope to share what I learned through this unexpected experience.

Building Collaboration

One of the first things I found out upon being introduced to the nursing home administrators and nursing staff is that they looked to me as an expert on the mental health issues of their residents. My experience suggests that while the nursing staff is well trained on topics related to physical health concerns, they feel much less confident when dealing with mental health issues. Similarly, the physicians attending residents in the nursing homes are experts in the field of geriatric medicine, but in my experience physicians are pleased to be able to make referrals for psychological evaluation of residents when there is concern about mental or emotional wellbeing.

For me this created an interesting dynamic. On the one hand, I was initially quite unsure of myself in this new environment; while on the other hand, the rest of the treatment and support team was immediately looking to me as an expert with answers and solutions. What developed was an attitude of collaboration. Realizing I did not have all the answers, I actively solicited input from the nursing staff and they seemed to appreciate my acknowledgment of their value as the primary caregivers. The mutual respect and teamwork proved to be a key ingredient for successful outcomes with the residents. The nursing staff served as eyes and ears during the week and could document for me behavioral observations related to my work with the residents. Similarly, I was able to write recommendations for the staff in my notes and suggest interventions the staff could implement during the week.

Building collaboration was, of course, equally important with the residents. Although the large majority of the residents I visited had no previous experience of psychotherapy, I encountered little difficulty in establishing a therapeutic alliance with most residents. However, there were some occasions where establishing collaboration was difficult. Many referrals for psychological or psychiatric services for residents came when the resident was demonstrating a troubling behavior for staff. In these instances, the mental health professional becomes a sort of behavior cop who is called in when a resident is behaving badly.

While behavioral disturbances generally are an appropriate reason for the nursing staff to make a referral, it can put the psychologist in a difficult situation, especially once word has spread throughout the facility that the psychologist comes to see you when you have been "acting-up." Residents are less willing to talk to a psychologist if they perceive they are in trouble with the staff and see the psychologist's visits as some sort of punishment. The easiest way to prevent this dynamic from occurring is for the staff to be proactive in making referrals, so that the psychologist can evaluate and begin treatment before the resident is "in trouble." Otherwise, it is necessary for the psychologist to assure the resident that the psychologist's role is to assist the resident and to improve their overall wellbeing.

In the most difficult cases, where residents expressed skepticism over what they would gain from visiting with a psychologist, I found it useful to explain how their mental well-being is related to their physical health. Some residents struggled to identify their symptoms as related to emotional or mental disturbances. Educating residents, for example, on how insomnia and reduced appetite are not just consequences of aging, but may be related to depression or anxiety, helped them to reconceptualize their symptoms and gave them hope of improvement.

In order for nursing home residents to maintain healthy living, it is important they maintain health-promoting behaviors, but mental health issues can complicate treatment of physical health concerns. For example, the loss of motivation and initiative associated with depression can contribute to a resident not wanting to participate in rehabilitative therapies, such as physical, occupational, or speech therapy. In some cases the apathy associated with depression leads to noticeable declines in self-care behavior and poor personal hygiene, which can contribute to infections and other physical health problems. Additionally, depressed residents often withdraw from or avoid organized social activities which would otherwise provide cognitive stimulation and opportunities for fellowship with other residents and staff. Furthermore, the loss of appetite often associated with depression, when severe, can contribute to physical weakness and lead to further physical decline. Early intervention is possible when all members of the treatment team are educated on the benefits of an integrated approach to care which monitors not only the residents' physical health, but their emotional well-being and health-promoting behaviors.

The Two Primary Interventions

During my short two-year experience working in nursing home facilities, two of the more common reasons for referrals were for residents who were struggling to adjust to living in a nursing facility, and for residents who were suffering from cognitive impairment caused by dementia. Each individual reacts differently to the transition to a nursing facility. The evaluation of cognitive impairment is an especially important role for the psychologist working in a nursing home facility.

The transition to living in a nursing home, or even a residential care facility, marks a transition on many levels for the individual. I have observed one of the more difficult aspects of that transition to be the residents' adjustment to restrictions in freedom and responsibility imposed by the structure of the nursing facility. This restriction can be especially difficult for those residents who move from their home or an independent living arrangement to a skilled nursing unit. Typically, the residents who had been living at home enjoyed the freedom to organize their day as they wished. Then, rather abruptly, they find their day is scheduled; even the very basic daily tasks often taken for granted, are now regimented. All meals are served between certain hours. The daily menu is restricted. Baths and showers come on certain days and at the time of the staff's choosing.

It is easy to understand the importance of such a regimented schedule. With many residents to care for, the schedule assures each resident receives attention to their basic dietary and hygiene needs. Without the structure, it would be chaotic, but still it requires an adjustment on the part of the resident and results in a variety of reactions. Some residents exhibit symptoms of adjustment related depression, and this can contribute to complications and setbacks in their physical health, as discussed above.

When working with residents having difficulties adjusting to the regimented structure of a nursing home facility, I found it useful to help them identify things still under their control and to work with the nursing staff to amplify the residents' autonomy in those matters. Examples include the residents' freedom to choose what social activities they involve themselves in, such as chapel, Bingo, or concerts. The nursing staff recognized that participating in social activities was an important part of the overall well-being for residents, but increased involvement was most beneficial when the residents realized this need for themselves. Supportive therapeutic interventions while working to gradually increase the resident's involvement in organized social activity increased their feeling of connectedness and community and were often successful at easing their adjustment.

A second important intervention a psychologist offers residents in nursing facilities is through serving as an objective evaluator. Viewing objectification as a strength is strange coming from a clinician with a strong leaning toward humanistic therapies. However, residents and their families sometimes have questions that need objective answers. The most important of these are questions related to the level of care necessary to sustain quality in living. There are many variables that come to play, and sometimes a resident and/or their family is in such a deep denial about the level of cognitive impairment, that an objective third person is needed to provide an honest evaluation of the circumstances.

Reporting the findings of a cognitive evaluation, especially when the news is bad, required a delicate, yet straightforward approach. Initially, I approached these cases with some trepidation regarding how the family would react to my findings and recommendations. However, I learned that in most cases the family welcomed having an expert lay the facts out for them, even when the news was not what they hoped to hear. In some cases, dealing with dementia, and especially dementia of the Alzheimer's type, is more difficult for the resident's family than it is for the resident. When a diagnosis of Alzheimer's has been given, the family knows they will be bearing an increasingly heavy burden of responsibility as the disease progresses. Families rely on the psychologist's findings in these cases to make determinations about living arrangements and the activation of durable power of attorney or guardianships.

Interruptions and Goodbyes

The relationship between psychologist and client is not intended to last forever. Every initial evaluation for treatment hints that there will be an ending. When the psychologist is formulating the initial treatment plan, they are at some level considering the end of the therapeutic relationship. The treatment goals are indicators of what is to be accomplished before the relationship ends. When the psychologist and client are discussing these goals, the two are discussing what they want to accomplish in their limited time together. There is an implicit understating that their time together is finite.

In nursing home facilities, there are many things that interrupt the treatment plan. Residents may face physical illnesses and physical impairments which hinder treatment temporarily, or require a complete change in the course of therapy. A sudden serious deterioration, such as is the case when a resident suffers a stroke or bad fall, can be unsettling, not only for the resident, but for the psychologist as well.

More unsettling is the sudden absence of a resident. These events are reminders of the unpredictable side of nursing home work. Residents are absent suddenly for all kinds of reasons. Sometimes families decide to transition the resident to another facility. Or, in the case of rehabilitation facilities, the resident may be released sooner than anticipated. There are other unexpected absences that are harder to take, with the most prominent being when a resident has died. Death interrupts treatment plans in a finite way.

Of all the existential givens, death anxiety is amplified the greatest in nursing home facilities and it is important that psychologists working with nursing home residents attune to this dynamic. It has been interesting to observe how residents deal with and talk about death. Most residents I worked with were very comfortable talking about their death. It was not uncommon for me to hear residents say they are ready to die – and this did not mean they were suicidal. Talk of death panics some nursing home staff; a resident's mention of death is sometimes mistaken for suicidal thoughts. Suicide in the elderly is a very real concern and real suicidal ideation should be taken seriously with appropriate precautions. Whether talked about openly or not, death is on the mind of most nursing home residents, and a psychologist working in a nursing home should be prepared to work with death in a therapeutic manner.

In the last few weeks, I have been saying my good-byes in an intentional way. I am preparing for a transition in employment that requires relocation and means I will not be working in nursing home facilities, at least not in the foreseeable future. Residents in nursing homes are used to transitions. There is such a high rate of turnover amongst nursing home staff that residents become, or seem to become, accustomed to having familiar faces disappear and new faces appear. In fact, in just my two short years of nursing home work, I outlasted countless aides and floor-techs involved in the residents care.

I have not taken lightly my role as a consistent presence in the life of the residents I have been treating. In fact, there are about a half dozen residents who I had contact with during the entire two years of my work in the nursing facilities. I have been visiting them routinely to process their stressors, check on their coping resources, etc. They have gotten used to me and many of them anticipate my visits Many had difficulty forming close connections within the nursing home because everyone is always leaving, or at least that is how it seems to them. And for a few, I am just about the only contact they have with the world outside the nursing home walls.

The temporal aspect of our being is undeniable for those in nursing facilities. No relationships last forever, and few relationships seem to last very long in a nursing home. Many times over the past two years I have had to deal with residents leaving me. Now I am leaving them. That old questions comes back to me, "What am I doing here?" I wonder sometimes if I have done any real good. How do you measure success in an environment where all your clients are in a state of continuous gradual decline? Then the reality of the situation dawns on me, all of us who have reached adulthood are in a state of continuous gradual decline.

I have noticed an unfortunate tendency for me to devalue my work in the nursing homes because progress was not as easy to see as it was in my private practice work. But, what I have learned from my two years in the nursing homes is the nursing home residents and my private practice clients have more in common than I initially thought. So, what was I doing in the nursing homes? The same thing I was doing in my private practice, striving to help people live as well as possible.

Two Key Questions

Over time I noticed that I was not the only one asking the question, "What am I doing here?" Many of the residents I worked with were asking a version of that question themselves. Some seemed caught off-guard by the aging process, as if they never had entertained the idea that they would ever require the level of care they were now receiving, and they had a hard time understanding what they were doing in a nursing home. These were the residents who often showed poor adjustment and struggled with anger and depression as they maintained a stranglehold on their sense of independence. Other residents seemed to have an easier time accepting their aging, and for them the question turned from "What am I doing here?" to "What more can I be doing here?" Despite physical and/or cognitive limitations, these residents strove to find meaning in their life experiences and choose to live with intentionality. I came to have great admiration for these persistent residents who kept on living even when faced with the reality of declining physical health and mounting limitations.

Observing these fundamentally different approaches to aging caused me to consider how I will be when I reach my later years. I have learned from my short two years of nursing home work, that finding an answer to the question "What am I doing here?" is important at any age and any phase of life. It seems to me that those who are able to find purpose and meaning in their answer to this question, and who then live a life of intention, end up aging well. Living well and aging well seem to go hand-in-hand and I want to do both. So, I will keep asking those questions, "What am I doing here?" and "What more can I be doing here?"

8

Finding the Right Retirement Home

Fran Korb

My husband and I started our search for a retirement home about ten years before we figured we would be needing to move into one. At that time our lives were rich with the love of family; we lived near our children and grandchildren and were able to spend time with them often. And of course there was the delicious freedom of having our own place. We felt that we could not have asked for more. Yet we were aging and we knew that this freedom could come with a price we did not want to pay: We could become a burden to our children if we became physically incapable of caring for ourselves. Our family is essential to us and we certainly did not want to become such a burden. So we got to work looking for a retirement home that would suit us. Perhaps part of this process was the spirit of the gardener in us; we were planting seeds that would take ten years to mature, though we did not know this at the time.

We began our search as part of social outings. For instance, once on our annual journey to the Bach Music Festival in Monterey, we spontaneously decided to look at a couple of places. All of those we looked at had been recommended by friends or family. There were so many places to consider that those recommendations became quite important.. We had no health problems at the beginning of our search, so we had the luxury of looking at places without the urgency of having to move into one of them immediately. Looking back, I think this is a very good way to find the right home.

We also soon found out that many places we really liked had long waiting lists, some as long as five or even ten years before space would be available. So my first piece of advice to the next aging generation is to look for a retirement home while you are still young and healthy and put your name on several waiting lists. We received calls from several homes as soon as our names reached the top of their lists; we were not ready to move in, but our names stayed at the tops of those lists and the calls kept coming in, without any pressure, until we were ready. They became gentle reminders that we could move when we chose to do so. That sense of choice was very important to us.

One aspect of this search that we had not anticipated was the extent to which it was a clarification of our own values. My husband and I love to garden, listen to music, promote peace at every level, and connect with like-minded people. Nothing controversial in this, you might think, but the first community we visited in Monterey had a large picture of a former conservative president hanging prominently in one of the public areas and we suddenly realized that we would probably not be comfortable there. Retirement communities are like small villages where everyone knows about everyone else, where community standards regarding faith and ideals and politics can be clear and rigid, and that picture of this former president told us that we would not be welcome to express our values comfortably if we lived there.

On a more practical level, one of the primary concerns we faced was cost, and our search therefore required us to look carefully at all our assets. The longer we searched, the clearer it became that we would have to sell our home in order to be able to afford the sort of place where we felt we belonged. Being willing to give up your current home in order to obtain one more suited to your future needs is essential in this process.

Three more pieces of advice. First, look closely not only at what you have to pay to get into a home, but also at what you will have to pay monthly to stay there. Second, will the home accept Medicare as full payment if and when your funds run out? Third, retirement home licenses are always being reevaluated; when searching, always look closely at the licenses.

Also be aware that not all residences offer options for independent living, assisted living, and skilled nursing. You want to be sure that the one you choose offers continuing care, that is, one where you can move from independent to assisted living to skilled nursing in the same facility, and not have to find and move into yet another residence when your capability and energy for such things are waning.

Focused Searching

As our search continued with more focus, we realized that a primary concern was being near our children and grandchildren. Family is first for us and having easy access to them and them to us is of vital importance. So now we were looking for privacy, for community, for gardens, for like-minded people, for a deep respect for life and death, and for closeness to family. We knew this place would be our last home before we died and we wanted to choose carefully. We put the word out to as many friends and family as possible that we were looking for such a retirement home, and sure enough we began to hear that such places existed. The names we heard about from more than one source were the places we visited in earnest.

We looked at four places in the main city of Sonoma County, Santa Rosa. It is the largest city in the county, with the largest selection of retirement homes, and close to our children and grandchildren. There was one we really liked, but it did not have the option of continuing care. There were like-minded people, good care, and our own space, but the availability of continuous care on the same property was a priority for us. We did not want to have to commute to see each other if one of us needed continued care before the other.

At another place the director talked about the seniors as if they were children, infantilizing the residents. Another place was way too clean, with manicured lawns. Being clean and orderly are certainly important values, but I could not imagine myself staying clean to garden! And another place required formal attire for dinner, which was not our way of living at all.

Then we walked into Friends House. Each little cottage had its own garden, not pristine and manicured, but in the process of becoming, as living gardens are. Not only that, but there was a great variety of gardens—Buddhist gardens, gardens with apple trees in the middle, gardens to look at, and gardens for getting your hands dirty. And everything was on one floor, and all the rooms looked out onto gardens. These gardens spoke to us of both the importance of the individual and the sense of community. There was plenty of space for individual expression and at the same time a strong sense of mutual support for shared, natural, peaceful values. No spotlessness, no fancy clothes, just clean and neat enough, and comfortable; a place to live and die in.

Consistent with this, the staff at Friends House were friendly and sincere. We were shown around by both an administrator and a resident, letting us see two sides of the retirement experience there. The resident showed us her own apartment and shared her experience of living in the community. She told us, among other things, that on Tuesday and Thursday evenings there was always an interesting speaker to discuss homelessness or political topics or offer a mind-expanding lecture, and also very good music on Wednesday afternoon or evening or Sunday night. We knew a friend who played some of that music with his jazz band twice a year and he sang the praises of Friends House. We knew we had found our home.

We decided to put our names on the waiting list. Every year they would send us a letter asking if we still wanted to move in and when we said yes that would move us up on the list. When my husband was diagnosed with Parkinson's disease it became clear to us that I could no longer care for him outside a community. It was at this point that we told Friends House that we were ready to join them and we got in within six months.

Admissions

First, we had to appear before an admissions committee composed of residents and staff. I remember being scared. Would I say the right things? Could I say I was a Democrat? I knew that Quakers were for peace, so political activism was probably acceptable. We told them we were involved in peace movements and that was fine with them. The last question was, "Have you applied to other places?" My husband replied, "No, we've put all our begs in one askit!" They cracked up! My husband was a punster.

We had to answer another important question: "If you are told by the director or head of resident services that you need to go to assisted living, and we don't have room for you here, will you go?" We knew that saying no might mean not being accepted, so we said yes. This was a difficult decision. Assisted living here is often full, so we went to look at other assisted living facilities close by. If my husband had to go off-campus for care, I would need to ride my bicycle to one of these (neither of us wanted to drive). We decided that the bike ride would be possible, and that our concerns about assisted living should not get in the way of our joining the community.

We were then required to undergo a physical examination, which we passed, and our official acceptance came soon by telephone. We were ready and excited to enter this wonderful community. If I have a regret, it is that we did not come sooner to enjoy more of our years here together.

The entrance fee is high, but prorated, which means if you leave within a year you get a portion of your money back. Most people sell their houses to pay this fee. If you do not have a house to sell, then most likely you will have difficulty getting in, but if you do, it is a perfect choice. Once in, the monthly maintenance fee is $500–700 a month, and the total cost about $750. You only pay for PG&E, cable, and telephone; those are your three extra bills. Every apartment has "Pullman" kitchen, compact but complete, with a range or full stove, refrigerator, etc., self-sufficient and self-contained.

Cafeteria menus are posted each week. You can choose whether you want to go. A large salad is only $3.50, and you can either pay then or sign for it and be billed later. You can also invite guests. If you want dinner in your apartment, they will bring it for about $8. You do not pay for skilled nursing or assisted living unless and until you need it. At most other places, you pay for all three meals, whether you eat them or not, and even for care that you are not presently receiving, such as skilled nursing.

Getting Settled

Everybody here at Friends House is on some committee. You immediately become involved, much faster than if you were living in an apartment building or other residential facility. You are partly responsible for the place working and you quickly become more integrated into the community because you are expected to take some responsibility for it. My husband loves to sing and he joined the madrigal group, a group of eight to ten people who sing at different functions here.

I have always had my fingers in education so I became active in the education committee. Our home is very close to an elementary school, where a group of us volunteer in the classroom, and we can just walk there from here. Relationships are very crucial for humans of all ages and I have personally become a mentor to a young man who is standing just outside my home right now. He feels like a grandson to me and even calls me grandma. He has a challenging home life but a great big heart. When I started volunteering at the school, the principal said to me, "This kid is worth saving." And now it is summer, school is out, and here he is outside my cottage helping me, a win-win situation for both of us.

As volunteers, we go into the schools and do anything the teacher asks. One resident is from Guatemala; the first thing she did when she arrived was to start helping the Spanish-speaking kids. Another woman is a librarian and works in the resource room, helping students with reading. I work in a fourth-grade class. I like math, so I correct their math papers. The kids bring their papers to me and I work with them individually. There are about thirty-five children with no teacher's aide. Our committee also helps organize a big volunteer program in this K-6 school.

The sixth-graders have to do twenty hours of community service a year and they come here to the residence to fulfill this requirement. They push wheelchairs, read to those in assisted living, and they teach seniors how to play games on the computer. The biggest thing we did this year involved an essay contest sponsored by the Library Association of Sonoma County. The sixth graders had to interview a senior and then write an essay on what they had learned.

We announced to the residents that these interviews were going to happen and asked them to sign up. More people signed up than the number of interviews scheduled, which surprised me. I was not at all sure if the residents would want a sixth-grader taking up their time. In retrospect, I should not have been surprised.

I was in charge of organizing. We had 26 seniors and 52 sixth-graders, so two sixth-graders went to each apartment. The children were scared at first, since they did not know what to expect from the seniors, but they all walked out of the apartments smiling and saying things like, "She lived through the Depression," and "Did you know he was in the second World War?" They called the seniors by their first names and what was most gratifying to me is that they came back later to visit the seniors they had interviewed. At the end of the year, we held their sixth-grade graduation ceremony here on our beautiful outside lawn.

A couple of days before this we had a picnic where the kids read their interviews to the seniors and two of the kids won prizes for their essays on a couple they had interviewed. This couple had lived together for 27 years but never married. They came here to Friends House together at ages 90 and 94, decided it was time to get married, and had the ceremony here. They said their vows and exchanged rings, a simple, Quaker-style wedding. Everyone was there. The bride wore a ring of roses in her hair. That was the couple the essay was written about. Some of the story was funny and all of it quite moving. There is already a group of residents who want to be interviewed next year!

I am having fun growing older. I am so happy to have this connection with the school, to experience this mutual exchange that is so beneficial for both the students and the seniors. At the moment my young pal is here, borrowing my bike to ride just for fun, and also to deliver some cardboard boxes for recycle. He is ten and a very responsible young man. I feel that I am cared for here, both in my physical and emotional needs.

"Clearing" and Religious Services

In terms of religion, almost half the people here are Quakers, although the director is not, nor am I. I believe in Quaker principles, but no one has asked us to become Quakers formally. One thing they all believe in is peace, not war, although some of the men here have been in war (and some in prison because they refused to serve). They do not limit their commitment to peace in time of war, however. They demonstrate it right here whenever conflict arises within the community. When someone is upset with someone else in the community, he or she can call a "clearing committee." I have been called to serve on such a committee in the past and it was a very positive experience, with witnesses to whatever miscommunication has occurred helping to clear it up. The clearing committee is not used often, however, since people are expected to resolve their differences on their own.

They have a Quaker meeting every Sunday morning and anyone can go who wants to. Every morning they also have a silent group meditation from 7:00–7:30. I consider myself a Buddhist, though not a very good one, but then I do not know what a good Buddhist is. There are also Catholics, Jews, Methodists, Unitarians, and others here, and we are all living and growing old together. Carpools are available to take you to the different religious services in the community.

Dying at the Residential Home

My husband's Parkinson's gradually got worse and eventually it became impossible for me to care for him alone. We got some help from a woman who came two hours a week. We found her through a list of trusted help they keep here. This extra help worked fine for a while but soon it became obvious my husband had gone into a state of dementia. I had two daughters here visiting one day and my husband had gone to bed for a nap. He had been in the bedroom for about two hours when I went in and discovered that he had torn the room apart. He said he had been standing there with Abe Lincoln, watching a crazy man turn this room upside down. I knew at that moment that my husband had to go into assisted living and it did not take long to get him into the assisted living facility that was a walkable seventy steps from the independent living facility. I never had to get into the car.

He received excellent care in spite of the fact he hated it and wanted to escape. Every day he had a new escape plan. One day he stuck an orange juice glass in one sock, a knife and fork in other. I walked in and asked, "What are you doing with that stuff in your socks?" He grabbed my arm and said, "I'm ready to escape! Let's go!" The sad part is I had to say no and he was really mad at me. He had never gotten mad at me before he went into dementia.

My husband hated this situation. He had to be tied to his bed and still he got out of it. He would climb over the railing and walk down the hall nude, saying to the nurses as he went by, "I'm leaving." The next day the nurses and I were laughing about this, yet it was sad how much he wanted to leave.

If we had wanted a priest or minister we were welcome to invite one, of any sort, but we did not. What was most important to us were the visits with the children and grandchildren. I remember one touching scene when our children and grandchildren took him outside the facility to the garden. He was quite out of it by this time. My son had written a letter to him; he was eleven when we married but became very close to his stepfather. He had written a letter that moved all of us and brought my husband back into clarity for a moment, with tears pouring down his face; he suddenly recognized everyone and told each of them he loved them. This spell of coherence lasted for about twenty minutes.

The day before he died my husband went into a state that I cannot even describe. The hospice nurse was there and said if he did not come back he would die. By the next morning he still had not come back but was still alive. We called his daughter. Several of my children and good friends were all with him. One of my daughters jumped into bed and hugged him. Then she held his feet and we all sang to him. It happened that day that there was a group practicing singing with those dying. They came in and we sang and sang with them.

Some were songs of love and one of the verses that still rings in my memory was, "I am holding you in love with hands cupped." The nurses came in one at a time and sang with us. We were all crying. My sixteen-year-old grandson was deeply moved. I held my husband's hand. It was hardest for his daughter. His son did not make it in time and I think that was difficult for him. It was a quiet, peaceful departure. We were with him all day. It was wonderful.

There was support for anything we wanted to do. This place has been a perfect choice. I am so happy here.

Home Alone

My life after my husband's death here has continued to feel supported. He has been dead two years and I remain active in the community. I lead groups once in a while. At first I led grieving groups and now these have become regular support groups. Residents come and get support for just about anything, including loss. One of the groups is on loss and aging. You know what they talk about? Giving up their driver's licenses! In one group everyone had given up their license. One participant was elated not to be driving and was so happy to take the bus. I let them talk about it and then they always end up laughing at each other. But as soon as someone says, "I want to give up my license so I don't run over a child," it sobers the group up and they realize the importance of not driving.

I have been teaching my young friend from school to take the bus with me. The other day we went on the bus to the swimming pool and had a great time. I am giving up my license in another month. I am 81 and feel ready to do this. My life is full right here. The resident coordinator and I get together and talk about all aspects of life. I can choose to be with people of all ages or not. I can have breakfast at home and at the salad bar for lunch. I use my bicycle to go shopping if I need to and sometimes my young friend brings me apples he has picked.

Support with Animals

A few months after my husband died, a cat showed up and it has been with me ever since. We did not have a pet when we first came here even though animals were accepted. When you have to move to the assisted living area your pets can go with you. That truly moved us. Everyone knows that the animals are important to them. Dogs have to be on leash, but they can go into any of the public rooms, the library, etc. They are asked politely not to get on the furniture. There are exercise classes three times a week and my neighbor's dog came to these. He slept under the desk. The dog was getting old, as we all are. One day he spit up in the lobby. The director came and told the owner that the dog could not come into the lobby anymore. In response, the dog peed on the director's leg.

My cat is now my full-time companion. I am grateful for our wonderful days at Friends House, aging together in serenity, in peace. We both enjoy nature, just as it is. The garden is not manicured, but full of weeds that I pull with hands blackened with earth. The cat shows me the simple beauty of the day and stays close by in this space filled with love and peace. I am grateful to this last home of my life's journey and wish others the very best in finding such a wonderful place for themselves.

9

Taking Care

Elizabeth Bugental

I sat in the park the other day, reveling in the green and the sky, relishing the quiet of my own breathing, the liquid sense of nothing needing to be done. Suddenly, splintering the silence, a stand of trees to my right began whirring and whispering, trembling the leaves into life. What appeared to be hundreds of pigeons and gulls, wings swishing, swept through the branches, splitting the sky over the treetops. Crowding the air, as if on cue, they careened toward a piece of green near the curb at the lawn's edge.

Their flight led me to an old woman struggling clumsily from a battered car, dragging behind her two bulging plastic bags. Dancing heavily from foot to foot, gradually upending the bags, she circled slowly round and round, bits of bread floating and flying in all directions like snow in the wind. Finally, her ceremonial dance ended, streamers of green plastic trailing from her hands, she raised her arms as if in blessing, her face suffused with joy, as the grateful creatures dived, falling and squealing, around her. Who is the giver here and who the taker?

This is the way I want it to be. When it is perfect, caregiving is like this, easily shifting between giving and taking, a steady circular stream, each gesture of help returning instantly in a pleasurable response, like making love. But, of course, like making love, it is not always that way. Every time I say, "I'm a full-time care-taker," I hope it is true, that I am remembering to take in as much as I put out. But "taking in" cannot be conferred from the outside, dropped in my lap. I have to see what I want and need and grab on. The energy and imagination has to come from me. That is the trick.

Waiting and Watching

Almost six years ago, my husband suffered a stroke. I woke up one morning to find our dog stretched next to his body on the bed, refusing to move. Usually, the minute I am awake, Dickens is racing to the door, impatient for me to dress and get him outside for his morning walk. But this morning, standing beside the bed, trying to talk to my husband who is muttering incoherently and unable to move most of his body, my fingers automatically dialing 911. I felt coldly numb. I fought to keep my brain working, to remember our address and phone number, to find the words to describe Jim's symptoms to the dispatcher. I fought to keep thinking coherently when the paramedics came pounding up the stairs, loaded Jim onto the stretcher, and carried him down to the ambulance. I remained coherent enough to call my daughter, then my friend Jean for support, then another friend to come get the dog. I felt disembodied as I dressed, figured out what I needed to take to the hospital—purse, wallet, Kaiser card, a book, an apple. I felt myself rushing in slow motion, aware every second that Jim was going ahead without me, that I needed to be at his side. Move, move, I could not move fast enough.

Then, abruptly, I must sit and wait. Emergency rooms—hospitals—are places of waiting. If you cannot wait, you cannot be there. If you have to be there, you have to wait. There is no other possibility. Sometimes you have to gently remind an overworked staff member that you are still there. Sometimes you have to take matters into your own hands to get something you need, but mostly you have to wait. Wait while blood is drawn and scans are completed and urine is tested, wait until the right doctor arrives to do the evaluation, wait while a bed is found in the hospital, wait while a course of treatment is decided upon, wait until the patient can be moved, wait while the patient is being moved, wait until you can talk with the doctor, wait until you can get into the room where he is, and then wait for days and days and days while he slowly recovers.

Waiting in hospitals, intensive care or rehab, is not passive. It often includes careful watching. Overworked, underpaid hospital workers have too much to do. They need help. If we can offer help in kindness and appreciation for their efforts, we can join the team and watch over our loved one. Is the intravenous bag empty, does he need to use the bedpan, does the catheter bag need emptying, did the aide bring the right food (he could choke with the wrong food), is the railing up on the bed, did he get his shower, is there a pillow between his legs, did they remember the thickened water, does he need another blanket?

More subtly, is he sad or depressed, does he need more company, less company, is he sleeping well, what is he trying to tell me, what can I do to make him feel better?

I have to be more assertive than is sometimes comfortable for me, insist on seeing the doctor when I think it important; go looking for a nurse or aide when I cannot take care of what Jim needs. Make myself a nuisance if I need help.

Even before he was home, I was already a caregiver. I began longing to have him completely under my own care, somewhere familiar where I could be in charge, where I did not have to leave at 9:30 p.m. and lie awake at home worrying that he, escape artist that he is, will try to climb out of bed as he has so many times, once forcing the staff to put his bed out in the hall at night so they could watch him.

The intensity of hospital waiting and watching is a preparation for the continuing W&W that is always a part of caregiving. It is the beginning of an education that will last as long as the job.

Taking in Care while Watching and Waiting

Letting Others Help

What do I need for this part of my job? And, if I can figure out what I need, can I let myself receive help, and if I receive, can I really take in the love that accompanies the giving when it is offered? Accepting help is only the first step. Beyond that, is allowing myself to realize that someone wishes to take care of me, and beyond that is the pleasure of being cared about so that appreciation is heartfelt and healing. This is necessary inner work if I wish to turn frustration and impatience into positive energy. Here are some things I have learned:

Bedside. My daughter and son-in-law sat by my husband's bed during the night on alternate days of the first week he was hospitalized. I trusted them with him and knew they were choosing to be there. But it was hard for me, hard to relinquish my post, hard to allow them to leave their own busy lives and jobs to be there. To resist their offer would be to miss a very loving message from them and cut them out of their rightful place in this crisis, and in fact, once I let them in, I felt less alone and more cared for. Others came during the day, giving me time to eat and rest and walk, go home and shower, nap, or just sit a little in the sun. Depending on how long they were able to stay, I could decide what I really needed for myself. My friend, John, made it all easier by creating a schedule so that when people offered to come I could suggest a time when no one else would be there. It is a simple idea, but if John had not offered to do it, I would not have thought of it. A whole crowd of people at once is not really a help and often leaves the patient more alone and fatigued than ever as they all visit with each other.

House care. Someone who wants to help can be asked to pick up mail and newspapers, water the yard, let the neighbors know what's going on. If we are working, someone from our workplace can do the same sorts of things there.

Food. Providing food for people in times of stress is an old-fashioned, time-tested way of being helpful. I never realized until I was a caregiver what a huge help it really is. After Jim was home I especially appreciated several friends dropping off delicious meals. But even during the watching and waiting part of the experience, when I could not think about food, I was grateful to have a smoothie slipped into my hand at the hospital or be given something to munch on all by myself later, in the middle of the night.

Communication. The phone, at home and in our pocket, is both a lifeline and a problem. When Jim was in rehab for three weeks, family and friends were calling frequently to ask how we were and what they could do to help. I wanted to hear their voices and take in the comfort that was being offered, but I could not manage the interruptions or spend all the time on the phone. So I put a message on each day, updating information and explaining how I was unable to return all the calls. I asked them to leave messages for me so I would know they called, and also to please understand if I did not return their calls. I also asked friends and family to relay messages to others so that they would know they were in the loop. I did the same periodically on email. If I had had a website it would have been even better.

Lastly, we can use our phone or computer to gather support, to feel the caring being offered, to initiate calls to the people who give us comfort, to speak the truth to them about our fears and worries, our hopes, our anxieties. Just as important, we need to remember that we are not required to take care of them, that this is a time to trust in their ability to take care of themselves.

Well-Being. Reaching inside ourselves to discern what we need in any moment takes focus and a moment of concentration. Maybe it is as simple as remembering to do some deep breathing. Or perhaps it is sitting alone in the sun, meditating, walking, going to a yoga class or the gym or the beauty salon. We can talk to a physician about a light sedative for sleep. During this stressful time any of these things may feel self-indulgent, but they are really necessary, not just for ourselves, but for our loved one. Coming back to the bedside refreshed means better attention and communication.

So all my attention was in some way focused on Jim. I was not sure he would live, and if he did, what condition he would be in. Often I felt outside my body, suspended, unable to ground myself. I needed both to take in care and to look inside myself. Yet often I would go into denial, "soldier on," respond vaguely or find myself feeling that offers of help almost as burdens, as though I had to please the person making the offer, to think of the right answer to their question. I now realize that anyone who wants to help will do so, one way or another, and having some specific needs in mind helps both of us. Those needs are different from person to person, but taking care means looking inside to feel what is really helpful and ask for it.

The Long Days of Care

Dealing with Fear and Anxiety

I know now why the words "icy" and "frozen" are so often used to describe fear. I was preparing our home for Jim's return and often felt as if I were handling things through a cake of ice, pushing through cold, resistant matter. My normal efficiency was reduced to a child's level, my mind split between the hospital where Jim was now, and home, where he would be in a few days. A bed needed to be ordered and moved into the living room, another bed moved down from upstairs for me; the right sheets, covers, and medical supplies put in place, furniture moved out, furniture moved in and arranged. I needed to phone for equipment, make sure the home visits were set up with the physical therapist, the occupational therapist, the dear lady who would come to bathe him several times a week. My team. Would they come? Would we get along?

But what really haunted me was the fear that he would have another stroke, this one even worse than the one before. What if I was asleep as I had been the last time? Would I dare sleep? What if he fell on his way to the bathroom? What if he just stopped breathing in the middle of the night?

Those fears and more have never left me. They were certainly heightened when I first brought Jim home, but they still go on. In the early days, thanks to Kaiser, I did have "my team" in place. Efficient and knowledgeable help is a necessity—someone to answer questions, to set up routines, to give ongoing advice.

I have learned that the best way to manage my fear is to constantly practice staying in the present moment, a lifelong endeavor that requires awareness, discipline, and concentration. As in meditation, the mind wanders, borrowing trouble from an unknown future, reading portents in everyday mental and bodily fluctuations. Whether we wish it or not, change will take place; and there are many unknowns ahead. The inner juggling act consists of making plans without anticipating disaster. On a daily level, I call this "conscious denial," and consider it a positive strategy. Although I know very well that Jim has little or no memory of our life together, I choose to live with him as if he has, and only when he brings it up do I stop to mourn with him over the years he has lost. At those moments I tell him, "I am holding the memories for both of us." As I talk with him, my fear dissipates because we are *just then* in the moment, dealing with the tragedy of his loss. I am with him as we mourn together. Fear has given way to intimacy.

My biggest fear, of course, is losing him. Probably he will die before I do, but I do not know that for sure. Even if I did, pulling away from fear would also pull me away from him, and I would miss the warmth of this final life-phase we are sharing.

I can also help myself by sharing this fear with my close friends, especially those who have lost their spouses and understand the immensity of this loss. Even their sadness is reassuring. If they are able to acknowledge their loss and ongoing grief, then I can find companionship in their validation of my feelings. With their encouragement, I am sometimes able to let go of the fear just enough to renew my gratitude for the precious time Jim and I still have together.

Sometimes our daughter says to me, "Okay, Mom, what's Plan B?" She means, have I taken care of all the contingencies, do I have a program in place for whatever comes next? And I usually answer something like, "I'm working on it," meaning that I'm taking little steps as they seem appropriate, to find more help, to scan possibilities if he becomes more incapacitated. But my style, which may not work for everyone, is to gather information more like a magpie than a computer. That is my way of keeping a balance between living in dread and hiding in denial. I am valuing the present more than the future since I can't possibly foresee everything that is ahead. And now I know I can count on myself to go into high gear when that unknown crisis is real. Perhaps most important of all, I've learned to yell for help.

Anger and Frustration

For me, perhaps because I am an older woman, fatigue is the enemy. When I am tired, usually in the late afternoon and evening, all my sub-personalities come out. I have even given them self-explanatory names: Betty Bitch, Susie Sullen, and Mary Martyr. I recognize them when they appear, but if I am tired they take on a life of their own. As I huff and explode around the house, my husband becomes a mere onlooker to a drama of my own making. Usually the things that annoy me in the afternoon are the same things that happened in the morning, which at that time did not seem terribly difficult and sometimes were even a source of amusement between us—I am answering the same question over and over, making conversation he does not quite hear and which I have to repeat until he does. Being more tired, I am even more likely to drop the groceries, lose my purse or my glasses, fall over the dog. Ordinary annoyances suddenly become huge and impossible burdens.

I need a nap. It is so simple and yet I often do not learn to rest when I feel tired. I habitually wait to do "just one more thing" before I finally collapse on the couch. Inevitably, I wait too long and cannot relax, or it has gotten late and Jim needs to use the bathroom or it's time to take food out of the oven or feed the dog or water the garden or phone the doctor. Or I do lie down but feel I must jump up to answer the phone or the doorbell. My anger mounts, the world is against me. Once the cycle begins, it's very hard to control.

The other kind of anger, the big anger—"Why did this happen to me?"—usually only happens in the midst of the small stuff, which is why it is so important to anticipate fatigue and deal with it before it gets too big. All I have to do is tell myself and, sometimes, Jim, "I need to rest now," to turn off the phone and fall on the bed or the couch. I am the only one who can make this happen. And if I have trouble sleeping at night, I am also the one who needs to get some help from my physician to get the night's rest I need.

Respite. It took me a while to acknowledge that there are many kinds of fatigue and many different solutions. I now take Jim to a senior day program three mornings a week so that I can be relieved, for a time, of having his well-being foremost in my consciousness. I also have people stay with him for a few hours at a time. At first, I found all this very hard to do. I felt I needed to be the one who took care of everything and it was hard to justify the expense when I can work for free. But, with the help of my friends and professionals, I have accepted the fact that he deserves to have me feeling good about being with him, which means that I need help. I am especially grateful to friends who take him out for a while or just come by for a visit.

I do several different things with this freed-up time, all of them necessary to my personal well-being. Some days I work for a non-profit, which I find energizing, and at other times I may take a walk, meet someone for lunch, plant some flowers, get a pedicure, sit in a coffee shop reading a book, or write a poem. The point is that just having some time is not enough. I also have to stay aware of my own needs in the moment, which are different from hour to hour and day to day. Sometimes I want to be busy, sometimes I want to be alone and unscheduled. Sometimes I want to meet a friend or talk with my sister on the phone.

The continuing temptation for me is to turn all my "free" time into chores and errands, to rush around and get everything done. Of course, plans have to be made ahead and spontaneity is not always possible, but imagining my "wants" ahead of time so as not to go automatically into "chore mode" has become a necessary skill.

Community Resources. There is no way to say strongly enough how important it is to know our community resources. I found that once I got help from one program, I was led easily and naturally to others. The simple act of opening a phone book, turning to the yellow pages, and looking under "Seniors" is all it takes to get started. Kindly voices on the other end of the phone respond personally and help set things in motion. Networking among friends and acquaintances can also be very valuable. And the internet abounds with information. I try to remember to write down suggestions. Memory often fails, especially in times of stress, and what is not needed today may be welcome tomorrow. Needs vary for different persons. A person with a large family and support system may have very different needs from someone more isolated. Major problems, like lack of money, transportation, and medical care may take longer to solve, but persistence can really pay off. Sometimes it's hard to find the energy and spirit to continue the search. Enlisting others in the task can make the difference between hope and despair.

Humor. When my husband calls me into the room to ask if I am his mother or his wife I can cry or I can laugh. If I choose to smile and remind him he's almost 90, he gets it, and neither of us is upset. The dramatist in me realizes it is a funny scene so why not play it for laughs? We have many opportunities for tears, but luckily Jim is often more ready to laugh than to cry. I joke with him and play (yes, more "conscious denial") so we can genuinely enjoy the moment. When we are in the car and he offers to drive, I could remind him sternly that he has no license and no insurance, but it feels better to joke about finally being able to take the wheel after all the years he has commandeered it. He agrees with me that if he does not remember something it is just as well that he "doesn't remember that he doesn't remember," and we laugh. I bless him daily for his ability to catch the humor in his daily trials.

Other caregivers are not so fortunate. When the patient undergoes a personality change or perhaps is simply abusive by nature, taking out his or her frustrations on the caregiver, the need for information, assistance, and respite becomes even more vital. Hiding that truth from others, out of embarrassment or shame, can really destroy any possibility of peace, exacerbating normal feelings of anger and frustration, and may even be physically and emotionally dangerous to both patient and caregiver.

Joy and Gratitude

As I write this, the news is filled with stories of the hurricane in Louisiana and Mississippi. People wait for water and food on rooftops. Children in Sudan are fleeing from rapists and murderers, and starving in Niger. When I sit with Jim looking at the pictures on television I see his eyes fill with tears. "How can they bear it?" he says. We are comfortable and safe. And most of all, we still have one another, family and friends, a new grandson to adore. For those who are not so fortunate, taking on the challenge of each day, moving consciously toward the light, is even more urgent.

When I ask people who are dealing with daily suffering how they manage to smile, more often than not the answer is, "What else can I do?" And as Jim has always said, "We play the hand we're dealt." What I have learned is that it is we who decide to play that hand with grace or without. Every day is filled with opportunities to be grateful, to enjoy beauty, to wonder at goodness. Our never-ending job is not just to take care, but to *take in* care, to notice it wherever it is available, to pay attention, to be grateful. We are the only ones who can move our eyes and ears and minds toward the beautiful. Paradoxically, illness and need can put joy into sharp focus.

Now if I sound like Pollyanna, so be it, but remember: Life is very short and getting shorter all the time; how do we want to live the moments we have left?

Part 4

Gifts of Wisdom:
Awakening to the Unknown

10

Reflections on Life, Dying, and Death[5]

Hobart F. "Red" Thomas
and Laura Michaels

Some Thoughts As I Age

What the hell are these "Golden Years"? I don't know what they are talking about. It is a piece of pseudo-wisdom, a myth. Sure, there are "golden moments" in these years, but I feel anxious and frustrated when I ask myself what has happened to this wondrous machine, this body of mine, once able to carry me everywhere with speed and efficiency. And what about those creative juices, now all but dried up, that used to stream effortlessly through me, providing me with an endless current of inventive skill and imagination? These days it is difficult for me to remember what I have just muttered.

All my life I have been very health-conscious, always able to carry my weight and then some. I used to experience a wondrous high through my body, enjoyed my physical workouts, did not punish myself but worked at a comfortable yet elevated level. It struck me in a painful way, after recently watching my younger neighbor jog away after a brief walk together, that I needed to learn to relinquish some of the things I took for granted about myself—my physical prowess for starters. So what do I call this, a total loss? No, but it sure is a loss of something! Those long runs I enjoyed every morning into my seventies are gone, and I miss them dreadfully.

I remember long ago, during conversations with friends, that I spoke as though I would live forever. Now, at 81, I can no longer do this, but am not yet at the point where I can accept being the full-time observer I have at times become, briefly, during meditation, the

---

[5] This chapter is comprised of interviews (2005) with Red Thomas and material added by Laura Michaels, who experienced Red's heart filled teaching during the interviews.

observer who can say, "this is what is, nothing more, nothing less, just what is."

During World War II, while flying as a navigator, I stayed sane by choosing to view war as a game and to see the exploding ships as a movie. I did not see men dying, just ships exploding. The year was 1944. I was twenty years of age and had the overwhelming responsibility of navigating the one hundred men in my squadron on thirty missions. It was up to me to plot our courses to avoid fortified areas and get safely to our targets. I was responsible for all our lives.

I remember writing a letter at that time to my parents, telling them not to worry about me, that I would be okay. All the while I lived with a hierarchy of fears, the greatest being that I would screw up and get others killed. Only next was the fear that I myself might get killed. Most of the missions were horrendous. Only one mission in thirty went as planned and I flew, literally, by the seat of my pants on the others.

As an aside, the only thing of value I ever learned from religion was prayer, but I have to admit that this got me through those missions. Yet I did not pray for our lives; I prayed for a clear head and for guidance to do what looked like the impossible. I learned a lot about myself and found I could do things I did not think I could. I went beyond my imagined self.

After completing those thirty missions, an officer offered me captain's bars to stay in the military. I could have signed the papers committing me to another tour, this time with rank, but I decided I was not that kind of hero. There was too much to lose—my girlfriend in the States, maybe my own life. I made a bet right then and there to go where the odds were in my favor and left the service.

Thinking back, I did not really fear death much and I did not really want to be a great hero. I only needed to do just enough. I would play the game, I thought, give it my best shot and let the chips fall where they might. I was very clear about this, that I was not out for glory. I would not trade that time in the war for anything, but when offered the chance to continue, I knew I would not go through it again for a million bucks. The war for me was over. I had played the game and now it was time for life.

I remember a few years ago, when I was having a colonoscopy, that the doctor who was examining me looked at my chart and found it hard to believe that I was ten years older than my body suggested. As he looked at me with surprise, I felt my old competitive streak rise up and I smiled with a sense of superiority and self-satisfaction. Even my doctors agreed that I was beating the game of aging.

Teaching and Music – Healing and Connecting

During the war, I was also interested in psychic research, specifically the studies William James had done as he worked tirelessly to discover if consciousness survives death. Whenever I had a break or could get some rest from navigating, I would find myself reading James. I felt I had found my soul mate and it was he who planted the seeds and formed the basis of my interest in psychology, which I went on to study at Stanford University after the war. As one might imagine, Stanford was not very supportive of psychic research, so I adhered to their formal program and received my doctorate in clinical psychology while keeping my psychic interests largely to myself.

After receiving that doctorate in 1951, I was hired as a professor of psychology at San Francisco State College. Ten years later, I accepted the position of chairman of the department of psychology at Sonoma State College, where I stayed until my retirement in 1992. It was during my forty-one years of teaching that I was able once again to take up my interest in non-mainstream psychology, not as a psychic researcher, but as co-founder and provost from 1970-1976 of the experimental School of Expressive Arts at Sonoma.

This interest in expressive arts grew out of my affiliation with the humanistic psychology movement of the 1960's. Those of us in that movement, including such luminaries as Abraham Maslow, Carl Rogers, James Bugental, and Anthony Sutich, had, I believed, access to the techniques and knowledge to create a utopia on this plane. We knew, after all, that what the world really needed was love! So I set out, through encounter groups, to teach my students a Utopian way of expressing themselves, of connecting with each other, and found a level of love far greater in these groups than anything outside the human relations laboratory. I felt that my colleagues and I had grasped a very important principle—how to create love, agape, right here on earth and this seemed to me, in the end, much more important than research into psychic phenomena.

Throughout my years as a professor, I worked with Joe and Jane Wheelwright, two Jungian analysts, who helped me foster a much deeper relationship with my soul and increase my understanding of spirituality. During this time, I felt the wounds of war healing, and Joe and Jane made it possible for me to feel more confident about who I was and why I was here. Although I courted the idea of becoming a Jungian analyst like them, I came to feel that such a role was not for me. I did not need to emulate Joe just because I admired him and learned so much from him. Still, if I were marooned on a desert island and could have only one person with me, it would be Joe.

Which brings me to the second major theme in my life after psychology: music. In addition to being a spiritual and psychological teacher, Joe was a jazz musician like me, and I also have many wonderful memories of him and me sharing music together. I have been in love with music since I was six and I especially came to love jazz, which provides me with another way of relating to people. I always feel at home and safe from loneliness when I walk into a jazz bar, and jazz was particularly important to me when, as my wife got older, it became necessary to place her in an assisted living facility, where she has lived for several months. Every day I feel our separation deeply and find that my music increasingly takes on the role of keeping my spirit alive. I now spend as much time as I can playing music for the residents at her facility, as well as at other senior centers in Sonoma County. The light that music brings to their eyes also brings great joy to my spirit.

Lessons in Living and Dying

I want to tell you about my first conscious realization that people die. It happened when I was three or four years old, I cannot remember exactly. We were in the back seat of our car, my mother and I, and I was sitting on her lap. In that moment, I realized that my mother could die. I did not really know what this would mean for me then, the abandonment and loss I would be sure to feel, but I somehow knew that she could be taken from me and that this would be significant. Years later, at the age of ten, I found my whole world collapsing when my dog Pal actually did die. His death was so painful for me that I remember thinking, "If it is this painful when my dog dies, what will it be like when my mother dies?"

Pal's death was the end of my innocence regarding death and I quickly went on to realize that, in fact, nothing was permanent. Shortly after Pal died, my parents got me a new dog and I found myself emotionally attached to him within a month. My love for him was not the same as it was for Pal and did not have a chance to develop because he ended up disobeying me and getting hit by a car. I was so angry at him that I did not even mourn him. As I grow older, I find myself wondering who will miss me as much as I missed Pal?

Now, in the winter of my life, I face new challenges each day. What is important to me is not to waste any of these last days. I try, even with the daily aches and pains, to reacquaint myself with old friends like my soul mate, William James. I am not surprised in my elder years that my enthusiasm for James's work, centered on different forms of consciousness both during and after life, has never waned.

This year also marks the 35th anniversary of the founding of the School of Expressive Arts. A reunion of all my colleagues, students, and support staff is being organized. It satisfies me greatly to know I will get to meet with old friends and ask them about their lives and what impact, if any, expressive arts had on the unfolding of their lives.

When I think of how I want to be remembered, I regret that I have not transmitted more of what I have learned to my students (and everyone else). What I want them all to remember, I think, is that I practiced what I preached, walked my talk, and wanted most of all to be helpful to them. I also want the many professors who co-facilitated groups with me, and my many students, to remember the importance of music in my life. They knew it was my greatest love, and I hope they understood me better because of it. I still keep the music in me alive and I now look to each day that life gives me, no longer so much as a game, but as a way to grow and give to others the one gift I have left to give, my music.

11

Spirituality of Aging – Stirring the Spirit

Karuna Gerstein

In the short time I have been on this planet, I have had the honor to learn from many wise and remarkable elders. Whether simple or profound, all their advice has given me grist for the mill of my life process. Many of these teachers have said in one form or another that we are not human beings on a spiritual path, but spiritual beings on a human path. For me, this observation is liberating and helps me to understand that the struggles I experience every day are often due to the "humanness" of this particular spiritual life. It is comforting and useful to recognize all of the trappings that catch me – all of the things that contribute to feeling hopeless and overwhelming with "shoulds" and "what ifs"; and all the ways in which I knowingly and unknowingly make this life more difficult, all these trappings are due to what is often called "the human condition." In this human condition, these difficulties are not an appraisal of who I truly am, my deeper self – my spirit or soul. That "part" is perfect and unchanging and I can always access my deeper self (at any age) for comfort, for support, and for the inherent wisdom about who I am. Some call that part God, Allah, Buddha, Mother, Creator, Christ, Love, Divine, Higher Power, Lord, Jesus, Om, Great Spirit, One Soul, Energy, Light – all these names for me lead to the same place, that which does not die or leave, but is a deeper part of myself and each of us, that makes us whole and complete. It is what we all share and it is what in fact connects all of us regardless of age.

What my experience with elders has taught me is that as we age, we have an opportunity to continue to explore this part – our souls, our spiritual selves – more deeply with the benefit of life experience and, if we allow, with the curiosity of a child. I have been inspired to see, by some amazing examples that I can continue to learn about myself (in turn learning about and connecting to each other) in ways that encourage each of us to enter into this last part of our lives and gather the many gifts offered. Finally, these elders have shown me that my own spiritual exploration can continue and that I, like many elders now, have the opportunity to give the gift of the wisdom gained in this process; we all can realize we are wise and wonderful beyond what this human life may represent.

The Way It Is

There's a thread you follow.
It goes among things that change.
But it doesn't change.
People wonder about what you are pursuing.
You have to explain about the thread.
But it is hard for others to see.
While you hold it you can't get lost.
Tragedies happen; people get hurt or die; and you suffer and
        get old.
Nothing you do can stop time's unfolding.
You don't ever let go of the thread.
                    – William Stafford (1998, p. 42)

Aging can afford us time to explore the deeper values that have guided us in our lives. Time to re-new, re-tool, or re-fine our values and perhaps pass them along to others who follow.

As we age, we have the opportunity to tap into the wisdom we have and continue to acquire and allow ourselves to open to deeper meanings in our lives as we leave jobs, move, change, and face death. Each unique chapter of our aging offers us spiritual opportunities and spiritual gifts that can be integrated to deepen our connections to ourselves, to each other, and to the Source, God, the Divine, or to that which is mysterious, unknowable, and unexplainable.

Cora[6] was a 76 year old woman whom I met while she was living in a beautiful assisted living environment. An Episcopalian by birth, she attended church through her marriage and the birth of her children. Now a widow and facing end-stage lung cancer, Cora wanted to explore the questions and feelings she had for most of her adult life – the nature of God, the palpable yet un-namable connection among all of us, the soul, death, and life after. She wanted to explore what life was presenting to her now. In each meeting with Cora, we discussed her questions. Always, she told stories about her life, her experiences, her

---

[6] Names of patients and family members have been changed to ensure privacy.

art, her family, her dreams, and what she had learned. She became more and more curious about the teachings and writings from other faith traditions – Hinduism, Buddhism, Judaism, and others. "What did these traditions have to say about the nature of God in us? What about death? How does one prepare? What is forgiveness?" Discovering the variety and similarity of the ideas across faiths, along with the wisdom she had already gained, provided her with some of the answers. The rest that was unanswered and unknowable in this life Cora accepted as it was, trusting that the deeper place within her would allow her peace to sit with the unanswerable. Cora asked me to teach her some simple meditations that could bring her into her Heart and help to calm her as her pain increased. She embraced this whole process of exploration with the excitement of a child and with patience, grace, and humility that comes from aging and trusting that the threads of her life were guiding her. Cora died very peacefully, with her daughters around her, remembering that peace was in her heart. One of the many things that Cora taught me was that we are never done learning, and our spirit can truly expand if given enough space.

Facing our most unanswered questions is perhaps the most difficult part of becoming aware of our aging. For most of us, including myself, each birthday can significantly emphasize the aging process with the emergence of more and more of these questions. However, I often take that time of year to re-evaluate my own life. What have I done? What have I not done yet? How did I get here? Where do I want to be next year, in five years, in ten years? How is my life different/similar than I expected? What does my life mean now? These questions begin to open that deeper part of myself, that part I always have access to – my soul, my spirit, the thread. Questions like ones of meaning and purpose come up at any age, and as we age "who am I now?" and "what is life about now?" can offer important spiritual lessons and are essential to explore, even if there is no immediate answer. It is necessary to allow all the questions to reveal themselves and to let ourselves ponder them, write about them, meditate on them, talk about them, and/or pray about them, because the act of engaging the questions and lessons presented by this engagement will feed our souls and enrich our lives. The exploration of these big questions; sitting with the unknown, and turning to the inner wisdom that is refined year by year is a spiritual endeavor that is worthy of our time and attention, at each birthday and in between. I have discovered in myself, and have witnessed in many elders, that engaging in this process of exploring the meaning of our lives, especially as we cope with the fact of our aging, offers our spirit and deepest part of ourselves the opportunity to continue to integrate the changing terrain of life, to work and prepare us for what is ahead.

I met a 76-year-old woman, Pam, who was taking care of her 107-year-old mother, Mary. Over 12 years Pam had faced and prepared for her mother's death (at least she thought she had prepared). Now, on hospice care, Mary was truly declining, her body weakening, but her spirit was getting stronger and preparing for the journey ahead. Mary had been preparing for this journey for a long time, but because of her dementia she could not convey her unique, slow inward journey to her daughter. Talking with Pam, I was able to explain the journey of her mother's spirit at that stage of her life. I told her about the way her mom was moving inward to "process" this stage and likely her whole life. Through the metaphoric language Mary was using, we knew she was working internally to get things in order and to prepare. Her apparent working to be ready for her passing; the slowing of speech; sleeping more often; not eating as much—all were indications of her inner journeying and that Mary was well on her way. Interestingly, Pam, a working RN, while curious about her mother's physical and spiritual process, began to talk about her own spiritual process while caring for her mother all these years. She talked about the (illusory) control she attempted to maintain over the care of her mother in the process of illness and dying, and of her own aging. I pointed out to Pam that when her mother died, Pam's identity would change. She would no longer be her mother's caregiver as she had been for many. She would be an "orphan" with both parents now gone. *She* would be the older generation, the elder in her family. What did this mean for her? How would/could she navigate this new terrain? What support did she have—family, friends, community, prayer, herself—that could help her sit with these questions while she grew into the answers and accepted the unknown qualities and depth of the process of exploration? These were the deep spiritual stirrings of aging that Pam was reluctantly ready to embrace, and continues to embrace, with grace, curiosity, fear, sadness, ambivalence and a myriad of other feelings, even after her mother's death.

Movement of Outer Focused and Inner Focused – Spiritual Practice

One thing I have found working with most elders, and especially those who are getting closer to the end of their lives, is that the spiritual process in aging is one that can have a cyclical, rhythmic flow, from inner focus and processing—quiet contemplation, prayer, meditation—

to outer focus and processing—talking, crying, yelling, physically moving, getting out of bed—and then back to an inner process.

In this rhythmic flow, many reach for a form or structure to help steady the journey, especially the inner journey. Any spiritual practice can help to do that. Spiritual practice allows our own rhythm of engagement to our inner and outer processes to take place with a greater sense of awareness, peace, presence, stability and fluidity. A spiritual practice allows us to be more present in our lives, so that each event, each moment can be lived with a greater sense of ourselves as active participants instead of observers or passive objects. A spiritual practice need not be a formal, time-consuming, complicated, or an expensive endeavor. The most basic spiritual practice is *attention*.

As social beings in this world, we must relate to the world, to people, to things that are outside of us, each day. We eat, breathe, poop, walk, sleep, hug, make love, cry, play, dance, listen, look, feel with our bodies and with our hearts, read, watch television, drive, laugh, smile, move, and just exist with the external world. Any of these activities, done with *attention* and *intention* to the observation of ourselves in the process (emotionally and spiritually), can become a spiritual practice. For example, we can pay attention to our body when we walk, slowing our pace, paying attention to what our feet feel like with each step – the toes, heel, instep. This simple exercise is a spiritual practice that allows us to focus on what our body feels like, bringing us into the present moment, and into what is happening right now, however subtle. When we allow ourselves to pay attention to this simple external activity of walking we also come to notice what happens internally—our thoughts and feelings during and after.

One of the most recognized spiritual practices is meditation. "What is meditation?" a curious student once asked. There are many "forms" of meditation that one can choose to "do." Simply, meditation is being present in the moment as it is happening. Reaching for a state where the internal chatter about ourselves, the other, or the world is noticed and quieted, in order to allow a more full experience of whatever is going on in any moment. Anything that can help you to pay more attention in each moment can be meditation. Even the above-described attention to walking is used as a meditation in several traditions, as is the simple act of breathing. Paying attention to what it feels like to breathe – what happens to chest, belly, arms. Are my shoulders tense? Release them. Are my legs uncomfortable? Get comfortable. What happens when I take a deep breath, in through my nose and let it out from my mouth? What happens if I do all of this with my eyes closed? Or open?

If you already have a spiritual practice that feeds you, great. If not, you can simply begin with a breath or walking meditation. There are lots of resources—books, tapes, online instructions—that can assist you in learning meditation from a variety of perspectives. I caution you to not get caught "in your head" with the resources. Let yourself, let your body, let your soul experience the meditation exercises first. Try to let go of whether or not you are doing it right. Just be with yourself in the moment(s) of practice. That is where you will find the gifts, the thread, again.

We Get by With a Little Help

If the Creator had meant for us
to figure out this life on our own
each of us would have been given our own planet.
- Richard Squeri, Jr. (2006)

After about two years of age, accepting help is something we all struggle with, resist, and often outright refuse (myself included). As we age, the progressive loss of our ability to do things ourselves—drive, shop, cook, pay bills, clean house, take medication—can be a slow decline into a place of relative helplessness where we may suddenly find ourselves isolated, sad, lonely, yet not willing to reach out for help because of embarrassment, pride, or finally, the inability to know how to reach, or where, or even what for. The rugged individualism that is a fundamental value in this country is highly overrated, most especially as we move into our later years. Asking for help should not be seen as a sign of weakness in men or women, yet we often judge those asking for help. More sadly, we judge ourselves when we ask for help. All this clouds our mourning for the slow loss of independence and the changing meaning of our lives. If we are no longer capable of the independence we have had for the majority of our lives, then who are we now? This is a huge spiritual question which we have to let ourselves be with for a long time, hoping and praying that if or when an answer reveals itself, we will find peace. Sometimes, there is no answer and we have to find peace in the not-knowing. Sometimes the spiritual lesson in this particular place comes from an answer we can give instead of an answer we may be waiting to receive.

Abe was in the military for 30 years and retired at the age of 47. He invented and built tools, built several homes, built three boats, created art, tended an organic garden, cooked for family and friends, took care of his ailing wife until she died, and gave more than a third of his post-retirement time to volunteering and helping those who could not help themselves. Now at the age of 85 he was dying of cancer and struggling with his inability to do the things he loved. He lived alone but it was clear he would not be able to do that for much longer. His sons and grandsons wanted so much to help him in whatever way they could. Abe was reluctant because he did not want to be a burden. He did not want his children to suffer what he imagined would be a heartache for them. He did not want to give up. Abe understood the progression of his illness and readily accepted his death and the help and comfort provided by hospice, but he did not want to give up his independence by having family care for him in the ways he had always taken care of himself and others. He didn't want to give up who he was.

While talking with Abe one day I asked him what he had felt when he was able to give so much of his time to others, when he built so many things, when he took care of his wife; Abe beamed. He told stories of the people he helped. He pulled out albums of pictures of the houses he built, the parties he gave, and the gardens he tended. He talked about what he had been able to give to his sons over the years, not just materially, but his counsel in a number of areas of their lives. He became tearful when talking about his wife and how he refused to place her in a nursing home because he wanted to take care of her. All these things gave him joy and a sense of purpose and of really making a difference. "Now," he said, "what good am I?"

I told to him that indeed he was losing his ability to do all those things, but that inability did not make him "bad" or worthless. In fact, I offered, he still had something very valuable to give, something very special and meaningful to his sons and grandsons. By allowing them to care for him, he would be giving them a beautiful gift. He would be giving them the opportunity to experience all the love, joy, and fulfillment of caring for their father and grandfather at a time when he needed them the most. He would be giving them the opportunity to experience what he had experienced when he was giving so much of himself. And that gift, I suggested, would be the most loving and special gift he could give his family now and one they would carry with them long after he is gone. Abe was able to move past his pride and reluctance and did eventually let his sons and grandsons care for him. Later, they told me they were very grateful for having the chance to care for Abe.

That is what we all can do for each other. We already know that in the times of great need our desire to give can almost feel like an ache, because we want so badly to make a difference. When we do – when we are chosen for the volunteer assignment, when we help the stranded motorist with a tire change, when we serve food at the soup kitchen, when we pick that name from the community Christmas tree and buy a gift for someone we do not know – we feel fulfillment, we feel we have been able to do something good in the world. I charge each of us to realize that our conscious choice to allow others to help *us* and give to *us* is an important gift we can give to them. It is truly the gift of life and the gift of connection. The spiritual gifts we gain from *receiving* are deep and will continue to be uncovered the more we practice and the more we age.

> ...for years I've been watching, waiting for old woman
> feeling lost and so alone, I've been watching --
> now I find her weaving, gathering the colours
> now I find her in myself...
> -- Anne Cameron (1981, p. 198)

As I move toward my elder years I feel blessed by such wondrous life-enhancing examples of many elders, giving me a glimpse of what and how my later years can be. However, I believe that our culture needs to evolve from the perspective that aging is a time to be delayed, avoided, feared, and defined by references of youth. Linking the aging process to the rightness or wrongness of how it is done sets all of us up for disappointment and feelings of failure. If I only look outside myself for the measuring stick of what my later years should be, then I miss a huge opportunity to harvest the distinctive inner wisdom I have cultivated throughout my years. Then I miss the opportunity to become an example to others of the richness of Elderhood. If I also reach within myself for the unique lessons and gifts I have acquired over my life, and take the time to explore those internal places that hold my most precious, perhaps most powerful experiences, then I can find that wise elder in myself.

Defining Elderhood each day, searching for, finding, contemplating, and hanging onto the thread of my deeper self; acknowledging the big questions of my life and holding them with respect for what they will teach me (with or without answers); paying attention to the delicate and subtle movements within me as I move about my external world; allowing myself be taken care of and loved; trusting the wisdom I know I have gained to guide me through this unfamiliar territory; and by being curious and open to new experiences (external and internal), I can find a measure of peace within the stirrings of my spirit along this human path of aging I share with others.

And perhaps, the peace I find within myself and can give to others with
be the peace that will truly change the world.

References

Cameron, A. (1981). *Daughter copper woman.* Madeira Park, BC:
        Harbour Publishing.
Squeri, R. (2006). We get by with a little help. Retrieved from
        http://www.flowingdragonswords.com
Stafford, W. (1998). *The way it is.* St. Paul, MN: Graywolf Press.

12

The Gift of Faith: Waiting on God

Bev Miller

In this chapter I share my personal and professional journey with various aspects of aging. A large part of that journey has to do with grief and with the faith I found to help me through my grief. The journey began with the death of my husband when he was 43-years-old, and with the challenges that followed. As with most young families, our focus was on raising our children, working hard, and taking some financial risks to build a business we hoped would make our family secure in the future. Then life took a sudden left turn. Our family and our plans changed dramatically and the future we had planned evaporated like a dream.

My professional experience with aging began about three years after my husband's death, when I began my work with Hospice of Petaluma. After my husband died, I prayed to God to get me through the extreme sense of loss and sadness and the challenges of single parenting and running a business while dealing with a financial crisis. I also asked God to show me what in the world He had in mind for my future and studied what scripture had to say about "waiting on God." This set me on the path toward hospice ministry in grief support services and also brought me a growing recognition of the challenges of aging—professionally through hearing the experiences of clients who came to hospice for grief support and more personally through the challenges of helping my own aging parents deal with the changes in their lives. All this deepened for me the faith which I will now elaborate.

Death and Faith

My first experience with death was when my grandfather died of cancer. I felt detached from his death; I had been close to him, but was not devastated when he died. I was 14-years-old and too focused on myself, on my friends, and my own little world.

My husband and I had discussed death. Twelve years before he died he underwent open-heart surgery. He was in his early thirties then, when such health problems were not expected. He passed out occasionally and would frequently come home very tired and go right to sleep. We thought this had to do with ulcers, before he had symptoms of heart trouble, but we had a growing sense of something more serious. We went to Pacific Medical Center in San Francisco where specialists determined that my husband had an aortic stenosis, possibly from rheumatic fever as child. They recommended open-heart surgery. Since our second child was due to be born soon, the doctor advised us to wait. She was born a few weeks later and two weeks after that he had his surgery that went well. His recovery was slow but normal.

Nevertheless, during this time I faced a crisis of faith. I had been raised Catholic and married in the Catholic Church. My approach to faith had been based on fear, on a need to always do the right things, but what I experienced during my crisis was the truth of God's grace, that nothing I did could earn me that grace, it is free. So I learned surrender, to work on God's time, not mine. For example, as my husband recovered we had a financial crisis; we were buying our home and there was little help available for our financial needs. I prayed, "Okay, God, I surrender this to you," and wonderful things happened. When we needed something, it was there in God's time. When a bill was due, somehow the money appeared. Many things like this happened. There were other trying times in those early years; our older child, age two, made it through surgery for lazy eye. I had surgery for some growths on my vocal chords and could not talk. Imagine having two small children and not being able to talk! Everyone came to our aid—family, friends, neighbors.

My life became a study in waiting and trusting God. I would ask Him questions like, "What are we supposed to do? What are you doing Lord?" These questions were usually answered, although sometimes much later, and my faith continued to grow. I don't know why I chose to turn toward God when so many in my situation would have turned away, but I did. By His grace I turned toward Him with both trust and deep curiosity.

This is not to say I was never angry. Certainly there were moments of anger and frustration, as can well be expected, sometimes the anger spurred me in a positive direction and other times did not turn out well. Once I was angry while driving and took the turn in my driveway so sharply that I hit our dog which caused more sadness for my children. There are some things I do not remember about those days and I consider this another blessing. It was like the pain of childbirth; you do not remember exactly how it happened except that it is over. What I did experience was the power of healing and I consider this to be the reality of aging and the grace of God. I also hold the twelve years between my husband's surgery and his death to be another form of God's grace. It would have been much harder if he had died soon after his surgery. Instead we had twelve years more years with him.

When he actually died it came as a surprise. We had planned a trip to London; the day before we left he was outside burning some brush, came inside, and said he did not feel well. I wanted to take him to the emergency room but he said no. We went to London and the day we got back, he went to bed with symptoms of a cold. At 2 a.m. I heard him hit the floor. I tried to do CPR and it did not work. To this day I do not know if I did the CPR correctly. I could not bring myself to read the autopsy report for a year, but when I did it said that his heart was enlarged. They did not know what exactly had happened, but said his heart was in very bad condition. He had had a physical a few months before, but nothing had showed up. His only medication was a blood thinner because of the artificial aortic valve.

In the years following his death I had to make decisions about whether to keep and manage our business or to sell it. I decided to keep the business and raise our two children the best I could. I experienced some very cruel responses from some known and some unknown people. Threats of various kinds emerged, some which involved my children and I believe were to force me to sell our business; big and smaller crises were common. It was at this time that I began to have headaches; although I did not see the connection at the time, I was converting all the stress into a physical symptom I could deal with rather than letting it all overwhelm me. Here was another form of grace, God protecting me, only giving me understanding of what I could handle one moment at a time. I believe that was true for me then and even at this present time. During all of that time continuing to pray about how God would use my experience as my life continued on.

I read about a Hospice caregiver training in the newspaper and in 1984 took the volunteer training; although I did not know how it would fit in; again, one step at a time. I did know I wanted to help those in grief. I had so much support from family, friends, church, and work and still I was struggling. So I had no clue how others would survive such a loss without such support. So my experiences of death and grief were going to be put to use through hospice.

Those seeking hospice services are assessed for what group and individual services they might need. If our services do not match their needs, we have extensive referral resources. A licensed staff member interviews each individual and presents the case to a team of grief staff and volunteer service providers. Individuals receive services based on what they have requested and what the hospice team determines most appropriate.

One of the myths about hospice service is that it is only for cancer patients. No matter what the disease, hospice may be an appropriate source of services when a cure is no longer possible. The major criterion for hospice services is that the patient is no longer receiving curative treatment, only palliative treatment to manage pain and symptoms.

Another myth is that a physician has to refer the patient. A patient can in fact self-refer. The patient can consult his or her physician to explore the option of hospice or else contact hospice directly. I encourage a direct consultation with hospice. Often these consultations can easily determine if and when the patient is ready for hospice services.

Comfort care after severe treatment can have a variety of outcomes. Hospice's goal is to improve the quality of the end of life. Occasionally people are discharged from hospice care when their condition stabilizes and death no longer seems immanent; In general, however, people are not referred soon enough to take full advantage of the care and services that hospice can provide. People receiving grief support after a death often report feeling they would have benefited more if they had received hospice services sooner.

Hospice provides care for the patient *and* family; the patient and family together are considered a unit of care. Hospice assesses what the patient needs and supports the family in caring for the patient. A team, including nurses, social workers, home health aides, chaplains and volunteers, provides care to both the patient and family in the form of physical, mental, emotional, spiritual and practical support.

Another major hospice service is grief support for the family after a death, as well as grief support services for the community at large. The deceased does not have to have been a hospice patient and the death could be from any cause.

Through all this it became clear to me that my education had never taught me about grief—its aspects, its course, its treatment. How does one create a supportive environment for expressing the feelings of grief? It is my experience both personally and professionally that grief gives rise to feelings of sadness, anger, guilt, and depression, and that it affects us mentally, physically, and spiritually. Often it is accompanied by intolerance, confusion, indecision, and physical exhaustion. I know now that there is much literature available on grief and dying, and am grateful that this literature keeps expanding so that others are able to understand it better and support those who are dealing with it.

I joined Hospice at a time when grief support services were expanding to the community. These services include one-to-one counseling by licensed staff, one-to-one peer support by trained volunteers, and group support for children, teens, and adults with emotional support and education about grief. We offer grief support and education to schools and businesses — in short, to anyone who wants it — and we are part of the community crisis response team.

We educate people about grief and loss because this education is sadly lacking in our culture. The grief we address can arise from any kind of loss or significant change. As human beings we experience loss after loss. If people have an understanding of grief and how it manifests after an experience of loss, they are prepared to mitigate reactions to their experiences of loss that might otherwise be devastating. I want to emphasize the importance of preparation through education.

Education does not prevent the experience of grief—which is an inevitable part of the human condition—but prepares an individual and family to recognize typical grief reactions and then be willing to accept and receive support in moving through grief. Education about grief helps people feel more choice in their experience of grief and their reaction to it.

Grief groups can be both educational and supportive. The basic adult grief group runs for eight weeks, with staff and/or trained volunteers leading one meeting a week for two and half hours. Hospice has developed a format that takes people gently through their personal grief work at the same time it provides education about grief. The meetings foster confidentiality, safety, and trust, preparing participants to tell the story of the person that died. The story includes both the life and death. Story-telling brings back a sense of balance to the life and death of the loved one. Participants find healing in remembering the whole of the person's existence, a life as well as the death that recently loomed so large.

Participants present the life and death of their deceased to the group through pictures, memorabilia, music, and whatever helps to bring that person's life to the group. This session is very moving and freeing for the bereaved. We make sure that over a period of several sessions everyone has a chance to share their story. This sharing bonds the group and often group members continue to meet and support each other after the eight weeks are over. The sharing with like-minded souls brings understanding and validation to the process of grief.

Our grief services also address past loss. Very often people come with a current loss and end up talking about losses that happened years ago. For a variety of reasons, they had not fully experienced these older losses. There is great value in exploring these in addition to the present loss. Our culture does not address the fundamental human experience of loss, so losses that have not been addressed and processed continue to build up. We have developed one-to-one and group support for children and teens and adults, plus special gatherings around holidays, including Mother's Day, and Father's Day, and other special occasions. All of these events support participants in expressing present and past losses.

I never read any of the literature on grief and dying during the twelve years after my husband's surgery, but I read a lot after his death and continue to do so. The most important book for me has been the Bible. Much of what is of value in the grief books I have read is to be found there; maybe this is just a reflection of how important my faith has been to me. People use many names for the soul and spirituality has many forms, both within and without an outward religious structure.

Spiritual Challenge

I was faced with a spiritual challenge with my mother's illness and death in 1996. At first the doctors were unable to determine why she was unable to swallow, but finally discovered that she had suffered a stroke. We were not sure she would survive. I asked the doctor, "What would you do if this were your mother?" He said since she was rallying he would put in a feeding tube and wait. Her memory had been getting worse for years and the stroke exacerbated the problem. After she was released from acute care to transitional care, she kept asking for food, not remembering that she was no longer able to swallow it.

I left the hospital for about an hour one day. When I returned I found a note on her door telling me to come to the nurse's station. They said, "Mrs. Cavallini has "expired." I detest this term! They did not want me to go into her room, but I did. As I was sitting with her body, I had a prompting to look into her mouth. I found there was food stuck to her pallet despite the sign that said NPO (the abbreviation of the Latin for "no food by mouth"). At first they denied that she had been fed, but the next day they did admitted that she had been given food and she choked to death.

I was angry. The hospital was cited but we decided not to pursue a lawsuit. We also decided that we did not want any publicity over the citation, although it took us some time to come to this agreement. My siblings and I had to work through differences, but we quickly came to the decision that the person who delivered the food tray should receive counseling and that the hospital would no longer use the initials NPO but spell out clearly, in English, "nothing by mouth." The hospital agreed.

I realized the challenge to me as one of realizing that regardless of whose responsibility it might be, death is part of our story and will come in its own time. What would have happened if Mom had lived? She would have gone home, forgotten she could not eat food, eaten something, aspirated, and died anyway. The grace in all this was that if she had died at home, on my Dad's watch, it would have been unbearable for him. I prefer to believe that God allowed it to happen in the hospital and that the young person "responsible" was in fact the agent of His grace as well as learning a hard lesson. At the same time—and I see the contradiction here—I do not condone what happened in the hospital, yet I see it as an essentially spiritual event.

Although my Dad's grief was deep, he was protected from something much worse. In Proverbs 3, verses five and six, we read, "Trust in the Lord with all your heart and lean not on your own understanding. In all your ways acknowledge Him and He will make your paths straight." I have no "understanding" about what happened to my mother, but I trust that it was, in the end, best for my father. And my prayer was and still is that the young person who served that food to my mother will also find something positive from it. I also feel that the event was a gift from my mother to future patients at that hospital, which is that this will not happen to them.

Giving Back through Faith

I have lead and organized grief groups since I started with hospice. Being with people in grief has been my training. My faith has brought me to these groups and sustained me. I offer people hope and sacred space where they have the freedom to do their own internal work. I believe in people's ability to work through and heal. That is what I offer — holding their hope until they have the strength and recognition to hold it themselves.

Now, as I awaken to my own aging, I am also awakening to other potentials. In nearly twenty-eight years of working with hospice I have only recently been able to work with those who have lost children. I realized, for example, I was fearful of providing groups on child loss, fearful that if I did too much work in that area that I might lose a child myself. I recognize this was magical thinking. Deciding to finally lead these groups was not so much a leap of faith, but responding to an inner guidance.

There were strong indicators that child loss groups were something we should be offering: deaths in the schools and individuals coming to us for help. It was the people who received this help who started the ball rolling. Was I inviting this to happen to me? No, I was once again stepping out in faith to do it. Now, when I hear parents' stories and the help they are receiving, they outweigh any fears I had. I have heard these parents say that they do not know how they would have gotten through the experience without this group support. How deeply connected people get and so quickly! Certainly there are many ways to deal with grief and I know that hospice groups are not the only ones. But I do know the healing power of this way and that this way is my calling, which I have willingly answered.

Gratitude

I have many mixed feelings about my sixty-eight years. I feel a lot of gratitude for my life on a daily basis. My conversation with myself is about being grateful and what I might have done differently, though this conversation is not tinged with regret. I sometimes wonder, "What would it have been like if....?" It might have been fun to get more formal education, yet I realize I could still do that. This conversation I hold with myself on aging is about reflecting and looking at my life from different angles. The bottom line is that I am grateful for my family, friends, my ministry, and my faith. God has really taken care of me. And my faith has deepened. I am grateful for my hard times. Most of my life is grace. I get picked up, dusted off, and continue on the path of living.

My path continues as a member of the Board of the International Institute for Humanistic Studies (IIHS). Its philosophy and mission speak to my heart and to my ministry of meeting human needs through hope, compassion, courage, resilience, and tolerance. IIHS allows me an opportunity to contribute in a variety of settings, particularly in its outreach to the aging population and those who care for them. Through my personal experience with grief and my professional experience with grief counseling, I have found faith and service to help me cope with my own aging, and through my faith and service, I find my journey filled with grace.[7]

---

[7] For an article posted in July of 2005 on the death of Cecily Saunders, see http://www.telegraph.co.uk/news/main.jhtml?view=DETAILS&grid=&targetRule=10&xml=/news/2005/07/15/db1501.xml.

13

Cancer Koan

Barbara Sapienza

All koans are barriers set up by the Buddhas and the patriarchs. It is impossible for the ordinary person to pass through them. If you want to pass through these barriers you must realize your own self nature. This is called self-realization or enlightenment, satori or kensho, in Japanese. When you once attain true self-realization these barriers disappear in an instant as though they were nothing but mirages; and you will find that from the very beginning you have always been in a world where there is neither inside or outside. This is what Gateless means. Therefore, all koans are impossible barriers for those who are unenlightened, but for the enlightened there is no gate at all. They can come and go quite freely. (Yamada, 2004, p. 2)

I read from *The Gateless Gate* by Koun Yamada (2004), wondering whether cancer is such a barrier set up by the Buddhas. In Zen literature we often see ten ox herding scenes depicting the progression toward self-realization. The ox refers to our true nature, the one that is hidden, covered by our familiar self. It is the habituated or familiar self. In the first five scenes we see the searching for the ox, followed by the traces, the seeing, and then the catching and taming of the ox. It is at the point of taming the ox that our true nature (the ox) and our familiar self get to know each other by tangling and roughhousing each other and, subsequently, overcoming the awkwardness of the initial meeting. After which, we see the man coming home on the ox's back: the ox forgotten; the man alone; the ox and the man both disappearing; returning to the origin; and returning to ordinary life again.

Of the ten ox herding scenes, taming the ox, speaks most clearly to my experience of cancer. I really cannot say exactly how it is a turning point in my life's journey, but I know that it is. I resonate deeply with the fifth scene where the man and the ox wrestle each other, tumbling and sweating, getting into it. Maybe even enjoying the struggle, having waited a long time for such an opportunity. Each touch the other, seemingly at odds, uncomfortable, and in defiance.

For me desolation initiates the encounter. Specifically, the news that comes in these words, "You have invasive breast cancer." They stop me and bring me to my animal nature that allows me to confront the wall that I have built around my familiar self. In the encounter I desperately hold tightly to all that was my life, all that is me. Almost a year after my cancer diagnosis I know that the wall has tumbled. I know that I am no longer able to hold on any more. The cement holding my wall together has dissolved and someone is standing amidst the debris of my former self.

The older woman, who is strong and beautiful, and in some ways impermeable has died. The fortress built of over sixty years of sunrises and sunsets is in shambles. The blues and reds and yellows color a somber gray. My decorations- baubles of success, ribbons of friends, gossamer dreams, and golden plans for old age ripe with good health and fortune and that final wish for a peaceful death escape me. Nothing is left.

Having been fortunate in my life, I am now pricked by the needles of the fairy tales. My body bears the stains of the warrior. No longer can I call to the precious gems and stones of life to keep me solid. Nor can I bathe in milk and honey, splash tanned skin in rose-petaled waters, or wear my silken hair once veneered in olive oil freely. My cashmere socks do not protect me. I feel the shards of life beneath them.

Prideful on my sixtieth birthday, I dared to think that I am in the prime of my life. I walked the Inca Trail a month before my cancer diagnosis, walking to heights above 14,000 feet. I traveled the steps up and down for more than thirty miles, and I even climbed the steps of purgatory. I traversed the heights of the gods with plants and flowers sweetening the air. I flew down the steps from the highest elevations like the great condor, while Quechuan women in richly woven sarapes of bright colors protected their precious babies strapped to their backs. They walked their wares over the steep and ancient trails of their ancestors in their sandaled feet next to my iron clad hiking boots. Together we walked and smiled amidst the wondrous snow covered peaks of the Andes. Intoxicated, I marveled at the sixty year old woman who soared among the gods breathing in the thin air.

I returned to San Francisco enriched, healthy, and ready to climb and descend more steps, ones that were compatible with my dreams, ones that were inspired by the blue Andes. Perhaps it was here that I first caught sight of the ox. If the ox is true nature, I certainly had had a glimpse of her beauty, her strength of mind and body in the Andes. I had seen her at her best. I had been in communion with the mountain, experienced the serenity of the sanctuario as the first rays of golden light spilled over into the sun court, feeling for a moment the magnificence of God in my stillness and aliveness. Yes, I had caught a glimpse of the ox, my familiar self is getting to know my true nature. Is it that easy?

Then, in the early morning I felt a twinge or was it a tweak in my left breast. If it were music it would be a trill. The trill led me to examine my breast. There in the lower left quadrant of my left breast was a mass of unusual texture. My heart skipped as my hand knew what to do. I palpated my breast. I raised my left hand above my head and began again. And again my writing hand stopped in the same place alighting on some kind of a knot, a gem, an immovable stone.

It was October 2005, the changing leaves made colored carpets over the California hills. Golden hills awaited the rain of winter. It was as nice a day as any to visit my doctor to schedule a mammogram. It was a familiar experience to me, having had my breasts clamped and squeezed, flattened, biopsied, and even once as a teenager I had had a lumpectomy for a benign cyst. My mammogram results came soon. The X-ray is clean, but the lump existed. An ultra sound determined the tissue that I had found, a biopsy defined the tumor. Days later I was sitting in the kitchen with my daughter-in law Valerie when the telephone rang. It was Dr. Cowan.

"Should I sit down?" I sat down on the edge of the sofa, to receive the news.

"You have invasive breast cancer," said Dr. Cowan. I repeated the finding to him. "Um, Um. It has spread unfortunately."

"It has spread. Yes, yes, you can tell Peter," I said to the doctor. Peter, my husband, is a surgeon who worked with Dr. Cowan. I knew that he already had suspected that I had cancer, having examined me himself, advising me to the follow-up. I wanted to be brave when Valerie asked for the details. And I started out that way, brave or stunned, repeating what the doctor had said about surgery, lymph node involvement, treatment.

"What does that mean?" she asked.

"I don't know,"

Then, I was in her arms crying, "I don't want any of this to be happening. I don't want to have extensive treatment if I'm going to die anyway. I don't want chemo and radiation, I don't want, I don't want. I don't want to die."

She held me in her arms as I blabbered and cried, rebelling against the steps ahead, focusing on my fears of pain and suffering, and leaving my loved ones prematurely.

Was this Training the OX? The wrestle, the struggle? With whom was I struggling? Was I fighting with God? I'd been betrayed. By whom? Where could I put the blame? The dreams the plans were broken now. I was broken. I was gone. I was no longer me. I was a disappeared. I died.

"I died," became my new mantra. I could not focus on the positive aspects of my cancer, that there is treatment and a likely cure. Reason escaped me. Hope flew away, as desolation prevailed. The dream had dissolved and there was nothing except the cries in the night. I was an infant, no an animal. My cries could scare the dead. Loud animal-like screams pierced the night, shattering the silence. I cried deeply rooted sounds; sounds that I had never let out. I did not know who it was that cried, having never emitted these sounds before, sounds of a pure being in pain, an animal, a coyote, a pig. My dear Peter held me, ushering me into blessed sleep. When I woke up I remembered that Barbara had died, that she had invasive breast cancer. Who are you? Where did the other go? The sobs cut deeply in the quiet night. Harsh throat sounds coveted the night. Groans that originated in the deep recesses of my body, as ancient as time itself, poured out of my being. When I listened I could hear sounds from Iraq, Rwanda, Afghanistan, New York City, the delivery rooms, the torture rooms - sounds of sheer bottomless sorrow, sorrow without an end. It was only when I began to relate to the Rwandans and the Iraqis, the others who suffered, could I feel peace. It is only when I cried so deeply, with such rawness could I feel connected with my essence.

The nightly bouts helped me get through the day when I walked upright in my daily activities of doctor appointments, laundry, and work and family responsibilities. Day after day, night after night, the ritual continued. I began to fear that the nightly roar would scare Peter away. I feared that my cries would shatter my house, but knew that my cries were my truth. The fight with the Ox. I searched for a place to hide and found a closet in a downstairs guest room. When I slipped inside the small space, I returned to the total darkness for which I had yearned. There amidst the shrouds of my deceased parents, my mother's gold lame dress and my father's judicial robe, I entered the tomb. I cried, heaving with the animal that was me, braying like a patient donkey, feeling the floor that held me. I was at last grateful for something, grateful to be alone with the anguish of my loss. Alone, yet communing with the sorrow of the world. Is this Man Alone in the ox herding story? Is this a glimpse of what will give me consolation in the time ahead? I don't know. I know nothing.

In general, hope eluded me, giving into the moment was my salvation. Every time I met someone I loved, I told her of my pain. Her expression of love brought me to my knees. We hugged and cried together. We were one. I began to know something of the empathy that would soften my heart and bring me through this. Blessed by my loved ones, I knew we were one. My pain united us. Their love comforted me. In the pain there was union. Empathy was the gift that allowed us to hold each other and sway and swoon over the news. Together we pondered the course of life's turns. Together we were desolate and in this desolation we comforted each other.

I showed up for surgery on a Monday morning, beginning the treatments with several doctors. A radiologist inserted a wire through my breast into which the nuclear medicine doctor would inject a blue dye that would guide my surgeon to the sentinel node. The injection demanded a warrior nature. The pain was exquisite, equaling other pain: childbirth, a punctured ear drum. My mind flew to the disappeareds of Argentines, the concentration camps, and Guantanamo Bay. I was connected to others. As a warrior in training I had entered the sacred passage as an initiate in the hero's journey. I reminded myself that I was blessed to be receiving the treatment of choice for breast cancer, administered by competent physicians while I bit my lip and said the St Francis Prayer, "Lord make me an instrument of your peace, where there is hatred let me sew love."

Both sides of the coin. I still wanted to blame, to curse the day, to give up, to refuse treatment, to be the brat. Barbara had died. Someone alien to me was in her place.

"What are you saying?" asked the eyes of friends who heard my cry, "I died. I'm gone. There is an empty place. The dreams are gone. You see? Sister Mary Neill, a Dominican spiritual director with whom I consulted, said that this was the place when Christ left the tomb, the empty place. As a non-practicing Roman Catholic I tested this metaphor. The empty tomb, the vigil of waiting, an unknown and dark time before the resurrection. Is this when the man and ox disappear in the Zen story. A friend gave me a poem by Hafiz, "Forgive the Dream," as a way of helping me.

All your images of winter
I see against your sky

> I understand the wounds
> that have not yet healed in you
>
> They exist
> Because God and love
> Have yet to become real enough To allow you to forgive
> The Dream (Hafiz, 1999, p. 125)

The search for the Ox began anew each moment traces of him appeared in the faces of my friends and children, my teachers. Margie, a fellow cancer patient and therapist, knew what I meant when I told her that I died. She said, "Yes, Margie died, too. And now I am free to be grateful for each day."

Around the rectangular table on the eighth floor of the hospital sat several women along with the group leader and a nurse. I sat down as the new comer. Elizabeth introduced me as a post-surgery cancer patient. I looked around at each woman. Meeting their eyes I knew I was in the company of the dearly beloved, who like me were vulnerable.

"Barbara, It's Louise," said the soft voiced woman. "Louise T. from the Haight Ashbury Clinic. We interned together in 1982."

I looked at the thin woman with sallow skin and no hair. I did not recognize her but I knew her eyes. "Louise, it's been so long," I said.

"Yes, and here we are!"

Genuine interest filled the air. The women were in various stages of treatment. They were younger than me and some had small children that concerned them. How are your children doing? How have you told them? These questions flooded me, taking me out of my own concerns. Some women were undergoing radiation treatments, other chemotherapy. For one woman the cancer had come back. For another, who had lost both her mother and sister to cancer, sheer terror seized her with a fear that she, too, would die from it. These brave initiates were with me in my initiation rite. We were in it together, making excruciatingly different and difficult personal choices about our treatments, answering questions that had no answers.

During the holidays my children, adult and grand kids, consoled me. It was and is the children mostly that I turned to get me through. They were my teachers. They knew how to be in the moment. They did not do well with the abstracts. I played with them and whenever I got far out there, they pulled me back. And we danced together, swirling our scarves and hands and feet in all directions.

After the holidays I turned to my Zafu, a newly received meditation pillow given to me by a friend Natasha. Going to the pillow I began as with a pet in training, I'd say, "Stay, sit. Stay. Stay. No, Barbara, stay." I sat to witness how I was churning inside out and upside down; how I was angry; how I was scared. Why me? Then I turned to Spirit Rock where I heard Sylvia Boorstein, a writer and a teacher, answer my question, "Why not you?" She spoke deeply to me. *Why not me? Am I not up to the task? Am I above the pain of life?*

I had lost my faith. I knew this when I entered the radiation treatment waiting room for the first time. Inside were many woman dressed in hospital gowns, waiting to be called into the inner sanctum to receive their radiation, another of the many vigils. We did not look into each other's eyes at first. We were all lost in ourselves or just lost souls together. I picked up a little red diary and began to read, "El Senor, Gracias for not giving me more that I can take. Thank you, God, for your gifts. Fall down 7, get up 8." They went on in this vain page after page. I was dumbfounded by these words of gratitude for I had felt no gratitude for the gift of cancer, nor had I prayed to ask for help to give thanks. For what? I had been angry and blaming.

I realized I was in the midst of a crisis of faith. Cancer had brought me to my knees. I had not turned to my God to help me or to give thanks as these women had. Only had I used the St. Francis Prayer as a meditation when they injected dye into my breast, when I needed soothing words. When I learned after radiation treatment that I did not need chemotherapy, I was grateful. I had been spared chemo, unlike some of my dear younger sisters, who were suffering the toxic effects of their drugs.

Where do I turn to find my faith? Sylvia Boorstein at Spirit Rock gave me the name of a colleague and friend who did spiritual direction. Mary Neill, a seventy five year old Dominican nun, agreed to work with me.

"What consoles you?" Mary asked the first day I met her.

"My grand children, Milla and Isa, console me." I began to think about consolations and desolations - the trees, the birds, the others in pain.

"Do you pray?" I did not answer. I recoiled.

"Barbara, did you ask God to help you when you got cancer?"

"No, I didn't pray to God. If anything I was angry with him."

"Oh, you blamed God," she said as matter of fact.

"Maybe, not specifically, but I'm not in the habit of asking God to help me."

"Oh, poor Barbara. Look," she said, "I want you to pray, even if you don't believe in it. Because prayer speaks to our reptilian brain not our logical mind. It works." I left my first meeting with my spiritual director armed with prayers and tapes and a notion about being a Seven and needing a Five.

She was trained in The Enneagram, a program based on the Seven Deadly Sins. She told me that as a Seven, a glutton, I wanted more and more to keep me from feeling trapped. As such, my grace would come when I was more like a Five, that is, when I turn toward solace and a more solitudinous life. A spark went off immediately. I remembered the closet and the solitude that helped me initially. Then, the pillow and the beginning meditation practice, and now she'd asked me to pray. I marveled that something inside me had led me to sit in silence and solace. Some inner resource had guided me and continued to lead me. I had found Sylvia, Mary, meditation. Is this the faith that I had been yearning for?

A phone message from Sister Mary after our first visit said, "Barbara, I love working with you. You are so giving. By the way, do you have someone who will pray with you? I recommend praying with a friend." I was stumped.

I prayed to my inner guide asking for help with my confusion. The words passed over me like a gentle butterfly wing:

> "It's confusing, Barbara. The last breath will be sweet. I love you and it's okay to have confusion or is it two words, con fusion. Solitary time will help. Don't make too many plans. Don't do everything yourself. Don't lose energy, conserve energy, truly conserve energy.
>
> I wonder if I have died. Yes, your way of giving and receiving will have to change. It will without too much effort, get out of the way. Think of the creative process as your inner guardian, your God. She will not let you down. Think of her. It doesn't matter how long you live, it is how you live, and whether you live in your moment. Do not worry about suffering; suffering is built in, a human necessity. It is the basis of life, not to be avoided. Do not waste time avoiding it, then you are not living. Embrace it."

I died and then everything was a gift. And so this journey begins, my journey that will take me home; that will take me to my ordinary self.

References

Hafiz (1999). *The gift: Poems by Hafiz* (D. Ladinsky, Trans.). New York:
    Penguin Compass.
Yamada, K. (2004). *The gateless gate*. Boston: Wisdom Publications.

14

A Practice for Aging-Impermanence:
An Interview with Palden Gyatso

Myrtle Heery

Have you ever been "new in the field?" I am having this experience as I age and come closer to the occurrence of death and dying. We often hear the expression "new in the field" in sports, politics, business, and education but we hardly ever hear it in connection with aging, death, and dying. In fact, until recently American culture has denied the subject of aging, death, and dying. Aging and death happen to other people, not to us. But in spite of denial, here I am aging, walking or stumbling on the road to death and dying.

I find the term "new in the field" perfect for my experience with aging, death, and dying. I am a Baby Boomer. I was born in 1946 and am entering my 60s with the largest population to ever do so. Probably like many other boomers, I am entering these years with a thirst for knowledge, eager for every new book on the topic, and acutely aware of those who are older than me. How are my elders aging and dying? I want to ask my elders about this over and over again. We are a generation known for curiosity, searching for meaning wherever it can possibly be found, and then shouting out what we have found as if we were the first to find such meanings. So be it for my motivation in gathering these authors for this book

I usually see clear markers for my experiences of being "new in the field." I recognize a marker when I am around someone who knows a lot more than I do about a particular field. In the fall of 2005, I recognized such a marker. I was attending a teaching with his Holiness the Dalai Lama and mustered up the courage to ask for an interview with him on the subject of aging, death, and dying. I received a most humble message from his secretary on my answering machine, saying that his Holiness hoped I would understand, but that his schedule was full and he would not be able to speak with me, and please to have compassion for his situation. My compassion flowed easily; I took refuge in the quiet knowledge that someone else would come forth for me to question on this topic.

Later that day I was riding down the escalator to the retreat when I saw a simple monk sitting at a table signing books. A most interesting man. He looked up and our eyes met. I knew intuitively that I would interview this man on aging, although consciously I knew nothing about him. I turned to my companion, a Buddhist nun, and asked, "Who is this monk?"

"Palden Gyatso." she said. "He spent thirty-three years in a Chinese prison."

"What?"

"The Chinese tortured him in prison; they tried to make him renounce his Buddhist beliefs and convert him to communism. The torture failed. He sustained his Buddhist beliefs and thirty-three years later walked out of prison an older and wiser man. He has written a book about his experiences. Do you want to get a copy?"

"Yes, and I would like to ask if I can interview him."

My friend helped me approach with a correct Buddhist attitude, i.e., ask humbly, wait patiently, and—most important—be detached from the outcome. I followed her instructions and stayed present to the moment as I asked for an interview with Palden Gyatso. In a few minutes the reply came. Yes, he would meet me in the lobby for an hour that evening.

That interview brought me to my knees—both figuratively *and* physically. I was humbled by the experience of true rather than imagined suffering. Not something that *might* happen when I grow old but something that actually happened to a fellow human being for thirty-three years, facing the possibility of death daily. In recalling this interview, I have the opportunity of choosing what to share first with you, the reader. As I so often experience in living, the end of my experience holds the greatest teaching—precious, moving, and often riveting. So first I will share my last question in that interview with Palden Gyatso.

"Do you have anything else you would like to share about aging, death, and dying?"

"My final thought is just like I said before. I went to prison when I was 28-years-old and when I came out I was 61-years-old, all gray hair. Since I was 61, I was released from prison and came to Dharmsala, India. Now I am 75, and every day there is more and more gray hair. I think acceptance rather than feeling guilt is one of the best ways to look at aging, death, and dying. There's no way out of it. Even though the whole world might say the sun rises in the west, the sun will not rise in the west. It will always rise in the east. They are completely fooling themselves. I say accept death, and people who are wealthy can write their will to non-government or non-profit organizations that are helping humanitarian causes. That will be a worthy act."

After a minute of silence the translator asked me if I had any other questions. I heard his voice in the distance and slowly summoned my one-word response, "No!" My questions had all been quieted.

As I looked deeply into the beautiful brown eyes of this monk, I felt a quiet descent into my being. A quiet where there were no words but the palpable presence of a shared moment. If the experience of acceptance can be transmitted from one human to another, so be it. I felt deeply accepting about aging, death, and dying. I could also feel my mind rapidly awakening into its normal fantasies about death and dying, such as missing the chance to see my child grow into adulthood, or holding my husband's hand as he dies—the list of what I would truly miss about this physical existence goes on and on. Yet simultaneously, I felt that this dear monk was allowing me to see the possibility of absolutely accepting my death in this present moment.

How is it to be inside of acceptance? I feel that one word best describes my experience: *quiet*. It seemed that gathering the material for this book and this interview were bringing me in one way or another into a state of quiet regarding aging, death, and dying. Perhaps each of us has experienced glimpses of such a quiet state. It gives rise to the central question for me: How do I return to living my life *and* simultaneously hold this quiet state regarding aging, death and dying?

The answer to my question came as Palden focused on the essentials of living: acceptance and compassion for others. Certainly one hears these tenets over and over in many religions and spiritual practices—Christianity, Judaism, Islam, and in this case, Buddhism: first, acceptance is the best way to approach the experience of aging, death, and dying; second, give some of your time and/or wealth to humanitarian causes as a form of selfless service.

Thoughts began to sweep through my mind, but I kept returning to a sharp awareness of Palden's quiet presence. He was not going anywhere. I was acutely aware of the difference in our minds as my tendency to cling and organize my outer world seemed to speed up in Palden's quiet presence. I was familiar with the concept of impermanence as a basic tenet in Buddhism and certainly I could verbalize what it meant, but I felt that detachment was the difference between me and Palden in this moment. I was beginning to cling to what was happening and Palden was letting our time together flow along like a stream of water. Earlier I had asked the following question:

"This concept of impermanence that the Buddhists have is not a common concept in our country. I am interested to know how the concept of impermanence can help the people in our country face aging?"

"You are right. In Buddhism, we practice a meditation on impermanence and change. Every day we try to contemplate how even things that seem permanent are always subject to change. The more prepared we are for change, the more we will accept that death is part of the process of life. Then living becomes an opportunity.

"You will be less terrified, since you have already planted the concept in your mind that all things are subject to decay; this kind of meditation in daily life helps."

Certainly this practice of meditation on impermanence sustained Palden in prison, facing the daily threat of death, as he clearly describes in his book:

> "When the Chinese made a roll call of prisoners and a prisoner had died, the monks would answer, 'The breath left him.' Of course the Chinese liked this answer very much as it implied no responsibility on the part of the new socialist society" (Gyatso, p. 84).

He describes many tortures in his book, the following overseen by a Chinese officer named Liao shows what he frequently faced.

"Do you confess?" asked Liao. "Do you?"

"The guards held my arms behind my back, tied them with a rope, then threw the end of the rope over a wooden beam. They pulled down on the rope, hoisting my arms up, wrenching them from their sockets. I screamed. I began to urinate uncontrollably.

And I could no longer hear anything beyond my own screaming and the thuds of the guards' fists landing on my body" (Gyatso, p. 68).

Knowing this experience from reading his book, I asked, "When you were in prison, did you have any fears of dying?

"No, I did not feel any fear of dying because I already knew I was going to die anyway. Instead, there was a time when I wanted to die instead of enduring the suffering. There were times where I pissed off the guard purposefully so he would hit me in the right spot so I could die instantly. In Tibet, suicide would be breaking a vow for a monk, but there are times when I wanted to be killed."

At this point in our interview I felt overwhelmed by these horrors and could not imagine how this man had lived to tell his story. I asked him, "What was most helpful when you were suffering?"

"I also held my suffering as nothing compared to the Buddhist hell realms. When I was tortured bare naked and they burned my skin, I thought of the hell realms where souls suffer year after year and eon after eon. My pain and suffering seemed shorter and minor in comparison. To remember those who are suffering more changes how one feels in looking at one's own suffering."

It was very clear to me that to keep this perspective before him while he was actually being tortured required a very disciplined mind; it required a *preparation* long before the event of suffering happens.

Then I asked: "In your life, you have suffered much and have observed much suffering. Many people who are dying suffer and have caregivers who also witness this suffering. Can you give any support or advice for those who are witnessing this suffering?"

Palden Gyatso replied, "I have witnessed many prisoners die, especially in the early 1960s. Seventy percent died of starvation and their last words to me were, 'If you ever survive, please do something to benefit our cost of freedom' (their dying for the freedom of Tibet). Even though they had loved ones, they never mentioned those loved ones' names. Perhaps they realized that the loss of their country is a far greater loss than the loss of one life. It is an acceptance of death because death is a part of life. I do not give advice but do keep your mind *prepared*.

"Last year when I was visiting New York City, there was a woman who was staying with her parents in Brooklyn and her father was 91. I saw that the father was walking with a walker and his body was deteriorating.

"When this old man was walking, I could see that he was proud and was holding on to permanence, but the next morning he died. The daughter called me. When I came in, the daughter, the wife and the brother were holding onto the dead body, crying. I held them and said, 'It is Okay, you should be happy that he lived this long; this is the path that we all are going to go, there is no escape from impermanence.' Then I started saying prayers for the dying, to release the consciousness from the body. Then I told the son and daughter to give the mother some rest, but they wanted to have their mother active, so there was fear and denial."

"So there's a lot of fear in dying?"

"Denial in this process. In Tibet we call it numbness, superstition, like pride that denies the fact, like saying that talking about death is a bad omen. But here, they are completely denying the fact as soon as we are born from the womb, we are caught in impermanence; we grow up and then gray hair comes, there's no escape from that. Cherish it and accept it."

"Some people in America when they are dying have guilt about things they didn't do right and feel bad about it. In your book you mention that the Chinese call the Tibetans who escaped from prison 'big guilty.' Could you address this whole concept of guilt and the Chinese using the word 'big guilty' (not accepting Chinese communism).

"Yes, guilt is unfortunate; it is unnecessary, and it is futile. Sometimes one has a sense of regret, a regret about hating something, or the thought 'I wish I had not done it like that.' That kind of thought is more indicative of purification, but guilt is futile. Guilt may occur in different cultures also, but in Buddhism it is not necessarily common."

"And in regret, what would you advise for people who have regret when they are dying?"

"In Buddhism, at the same time there is regret there is also some sort of acceptance that you've done something wrong. You regret that, but at the same time there's some resolve: 'I've been unkind to people, I was not very helpful, I will never do this again.' In Buddhism that time is regarded as the most crucial time because you have the most opportunity. You have the ability to transcend all your negativity at one time, because of one general regret that you've done such and such in your life. You feel tremendous humility and honest regret. That time is the most crucial opportunity, according to Tibetan Buddhism. That is why your consciousness is extra sharp at that time."

"Would this include the Chinese who tortured you, if they regretted torturing you?

"Yes, we are talking about people who have more awareness. That regret will definitely help them on their path to their next birth. For example, it will help those who tortured me, if they have some regret, but it depends on how they practice. The sooner they can realize that regret, the better."

"If I am with someone who's dying, as one of their caregivers, would it be advisable to encourage them to express their regrets?"

"Yes, it's helpful, especially if you're talking about it openly. I knew a man who became very rich, but when he was about to die he saw that he had a lot of money but could not take even one dollar. He was a smart man, so he wrote his will to give all his money to people who are engaged in peace work and humanitarian activity. This is a very noble act toward the end and shows his regret for actions he had not taken earlier in his life. Unfortunately, this kind of act is not in balance. Those who tortured me, if they have regret, it will help, but it depends on how they practice, on how soon they can realize that regret."

"The sooner the better?"

"Yes."

"When you were in prison, you tried to escape and said that when you saw a single star shining through a hole you knew you could escape. I'm curious if you perceive death like that."

"Yes."

"This is the exit. The spirit goes through that hole?"

"Yes."

Wisdom from experience, and mine is not so deep, although I do understand that through that hole you cannot take your physical body, your possessions, your loved ones, or so many of the other aspects of being human that we hold so dear and cling to so stubbornly. This realization can be daunting, but at the same time the journey of aging and dying prepares us for the split second of death—that star shining through the hole—and then for whatever we hold to be true after death to happen or not. I turn now to a quote from his Holiness the Dalai Lama for the Buddhist belief about existence after death:

> Buddhism is one of the spiritual traditions that believes in the continuation of mind after physical death and the theory of rebirth over many lifetimes. Although there are some differences among various traditions, Buddhism believes that rebirth is essentially self-created—rebirth is caused by the propelling forces of the continuation of mind under the influence of ignorance. Under the influence of ignorance, birth and death are out of control and come again and again. As long as the grosser levels of body and mind are still there, physical rebirth takes place. When gross impressions are gone and only the subtle body and subtle mind remain, we can no longer make a distinction between life, death, or birth in the ordinary sense. At this point, physical birth ends, but the subtle body and subtle mind remain until reaching nirvana. Nirvana, or enlightenment, means no more birth under influence of ignorance. So that's the Buddhist concept (big laugh)! (Rosen, 1998, p. 126)

The Buddhist explanation of existence after death has attracted Baby Boomers and many others. For many, this belief has become a solace concerning death. Neither his Holiness nor Palden Gyatso are advocating that we take up Buddhism. In fact, it is quite the opposite. They both encourage Westerners to return to the roots of their own religion and practices. Meditation on impermanence is not a departure from any religious belief or practice, but a practical preparation for the aging process, with an emphasis on preparation through practice. I will probably never know the experience of being exiled from my homeland or of being physically tortured for my beliefs. But I can be moved by these experiences and look with awe and respect upon those who have undergone them and now live in a deep state of awareness of impermanence.

In part, the easiest explanation of being drawn to meditation on impermanence is the simple fact that our daily aging gives us a continual experience of it. A very dear friend who lived to be 99 once told me something very wise: "Myrtle, as you age you will look in that mirror and ask with surprise, 'Myrtle, is that you?' The physical person in the mirror will be hard to recognize and accept."

My friend had never practiced meditation on impermanence but knew the truth of impermanence by looking in the mirror. The challenge lies in accepting and embracing this reality. Aging, death, and dying can be truly experienced as "golden years," and not just as a cliché, if we awaken to impermanence and embrace meditation on it as a daily practice.

His Holiness the Dalai Lama speaks humbly about his daily practice:

> The cornerstone of my own practice is reflection on the four basic teachings of impermanence, suffering, emptiness, and selflessness. In addition, as a part of eight different daily ritual practices, I meditate on the stages of dying. I imagine the dissolution of the earth element into water, the water element into fire, and so forth. Though I cannot report any profound experience, there is a little stoppage of breath when the ritual calls for imagining the dissolving of all appearances. I am sure more complete visions manifest if a practitioner visualizes the dissolutions in a more leisurely and thorough way. Since my daily practices of deity yoga all involve visualizing death, I am habituating myself to the process, and thus at the actual time of death these steps will supposedly be familiar. But whether I will succeed or not, I do not know. (Hopkins, 2002, pp. 162-163)

I am humbled to read of such dedication and discipline to practice, and was greatly humbled by meeting Palden Gyatso. Suffering is a great teacher of impermanence. Aging is often accompanied by physical, emotional, or spiritual suffering no matter where or who we are. We can very easily experience prison in our own minds, especially as our bodies and our faculties begin to let us down and keep us from enjoying the mobility and independence we once took for granted.

Entering the field of aging we all have choices, as Palden Gyatso has so courageously shown. We can resist the physical changes that time works on the body and the many losses that occur on all levels. Or we can accept them. Acceptance is not easy; true acceptance requires disciplined practice *before* the fact.

I want to thank Palden Gyatso for sharing his moving story, for being a teacher on this subject of aging with dignity and grace. He reminds me that through practice I can have control over my reactions to aging. How I react to the fact of impermanence is my choice. I hope that the sharings in this chapter will inspire you to undertake a disciplined practice of not only accepting impermanence as part of your journey of aging, death, and dying, but experiencing impermanence as an instrument for liberation.

In closing, I would like to share a somber answer His Holiness the Dalai Lama gave in 2005 to my public question: "There is denial in America about aging, death, and dying. What advise do you have?"

"Overcome denial. Of course, if one had lived a more realistic life these problems would not arise."

References

Gyatso, P. (1998). *The autobiography of a Tibetan monk* (T. Shakya, Trans.). New York: Grove Press.

Hopkins, J. (2002). *His Holiness the Dalai Lama: Advice on dying and living a better life.* New York: Atria Books.

Rosen, J. (1998). *Experiencing the soul.* Carlsbad, CA: Hay House.

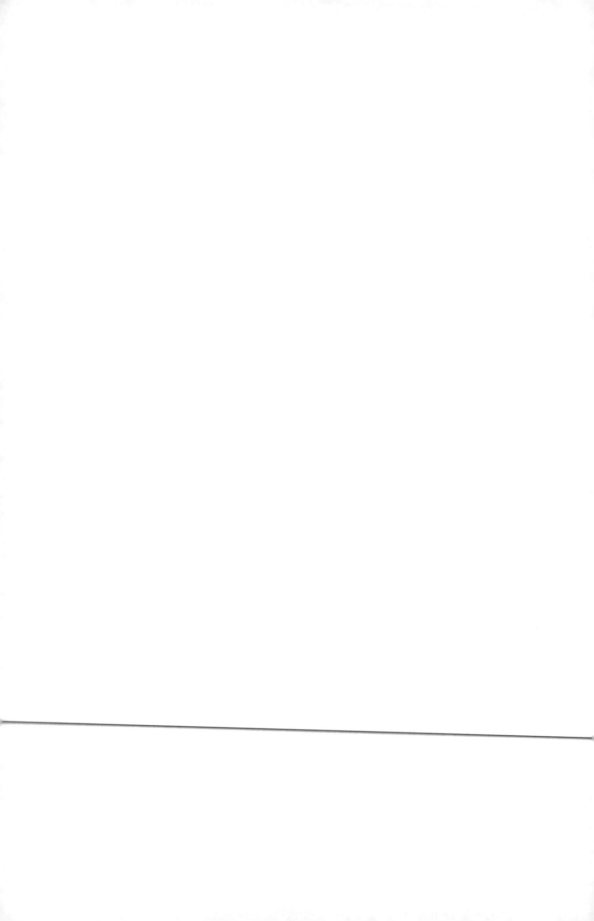

15

Growing Old

Carol Cook

Growing old is the price we pay
for living long

I'm beginning to feel it now
A slow, begrudging disengagement
From everything I have worked so hard to build

My home
My children
My career
My body
My intellectual capacities
My style of life

Sometimes I wish it had all succumbed in a sudden crash
Thereby saving me from these merciless realizations

But as I loosen the grip
on what I once believed could never be surrendered
I begin to feel the breath of spirit wafting
between these moments of earthly condition
And as I grieve their passing
I can hold more tenderly-- mindfully
to the fleeting moments of this precious life

And the time I once gave to holding things together
Can now be spent watching them move apart
Evolving somehow into wisdom
Allowing me to know ever more clearly
that the many forms giving structure to this life

Are but momentary glimpses
Of the true essence
Of creation

16

If You Live Long Enough

Myrtle Heery

Reading a book is a short part of our life's journey. Here we are now at the end of this short journey together, a little older and hopefully more awake to our journey into aging. Finishing this book is both an ending, and also a beginning — the beginning of bringing what you found useful in this book into your life.

On Edith's ninetieth birthday, we gathered by the bay to celebrate, to remember, and to receive. Edith was a granny to many, graciously sharing wisdom with everyone.

"Edith, how does it feel to be 90?"

"Well, when I look in the mirror I am always surprised and I ask, 'Is that you, Edith?' The person inside feels familiar, but the person in the mirror keeps surprising me. You will have this experience too if you live long enough." Edith gently tipped her head back and gave a generous laugh. Yes, generous of heart for those of us who still recognize ourselves in the mirror and know that we are also seeing ourselves in Edith in this moment.

"If you live long enough." These words awaken me again and again. What about not recognizing myself in the mirror? Or perhaps not even seeing myself in the mirror? And if I live long enough I will attend many memorials and funerals. I have lived long enough to look over the bay and remember Edith at her memorial. Edith died at age 99.

"And what advice do you have for us for living a long and healthy life?"

"Take a nap in the afternoon, not long, just fifteen or twenty minutes. And walk every day, every day. Start this discipline now while you are young."

"Anything else?"

"Oh, I am sure there is more but these two disciplines are what has worked for me."

I remember Edith, with her veins peeking through the thin skin on her hands. I remember the veins on my grandmother's hands and I see the veins on my own hands steadily showing more. My hands are like a faithful old clock, reminding me daily that I am aging. A little Botox or face-lift might temporarily stop my face from aging, but I remember pictures on the cover of a tabloid (called "adult comic books" by some) at the checkout counter of our local grocery. The photos showed the hands of famous actors against their face-lifted visages. The hands spoke the truth, with all the veins proudly proclaiming their age. The faces spoke of wanting what had been, and hoping for physical youth that was long gone.

If you live long enough a face-lift will drop from your list of concerns. Life has a way of throwing each of us challenges in aging which seem monumental and very unfair at times. When my husband was diagnosed with metastatic melanoma we were shocked. We felt young and we *were* young. My husband was fifty-one, I was forty-six, and our son was in kindergarten. We both aged with this diagnosis. My husband's hair turned completely gray after an MRI.

A panel of doctors at a research hospital told us about the health protocol that they had determined was best for my husband. I found his cancer a great challenge but that medical panel seemed an equally great challenge. The one female doctor on the panel was assigned to sit next to me and assure me with periodic pats on my knee that everything was alright. But everything was not alright. After several pats, I asked her to please sit with her male colleagues for the rest of my husband's protocol review; I was determined to ask questions no matter how many pats she gave me.

My husband sat in his underwear in the middle of a circle with all male doctors in white coats. One doctor started the questions to my husband.

"Where did you grow up?"

"I haven't; have you?"

One doctor covered his face while he laughed. Barely audible, I heard him say, "That is the best answer to that stupid question I have ever heard."

If you live long enough you will laugh harder and cry deeper. My husband was given three months to live and the medical panel recommended a neck section, removing part of his neck to prolong his life. We realized the doctors were only trying to give him a little more time with a neck section. The statistics of randomly dying on a California freeway and living with a neck section were literally neck and neck. He said no to the neck section.

It was a very scary time for us. Paradoxically, it was also a time of aliveness that I have never experienced since. It is a startling awakening to be told that you or the person closest to you is going to die. Death was no longer the shadow following us through our lives at a distance but was standing right in front of us and staring us down. The fact that my husband's body was sick and dying was the greatest gift of aging we have had. We woke up and faced the fears we were so used to denying.

First, there was the possibility that he would be dead in three months. Then other fears followed: Could he be healed and if so how and could we afford the healing of his body? And there was our son; how would we explain to a six year old that his father might be dead in three months? There were so many questions without answers. We soon learned that we were walking an unknown path. Yes, many professed to have walked this path before and offered answers to all these questions but none of their answers fit our situation. We soon learned that we had to walk this path as if we were studying and preparing for a very important school exam. We read, digested the information, sat alone quieting our fearful minds, and listened from within for direction. The reading gave us information and the listening from within gave us discernment and clarity of intent.

We decided to use a combination of alternative medications, to use our savings to pay for these medications, and to tell our son what we were facing.

The greatest challenge was keeping some distance on the fears that kept arising in our minds. We used meditation to distance ourselves from the rise and fall of unexpected fears. We began to experience the impermanence of emotional states, and quiet ourselves into the reality of death.

In the novel *The Art of Racing in the Rain*, by Garth Stein (2008), his character, Eve, is on her deathbed at the end of a long bout with cancer and speaks to her dog, Enzo.

"Do you see?" she asked. "I'm not afraid of it anymore. I wanted you with me before because I wanted you to protect me, but I'm not afraid of it anymore. Because it's not the end."...

She died that night. Her last breath took her soul, I saw it in my dream. I saw her soul leave her body as she exhaled, and then she had no more needs, no more reason; she was released from her body, and, being released, she continued her journey elsewhere, high in the firmament where soul material gathers and plays out all the dream and joys of which we temporal beings can barely conceive, all the things that are beyond our comprehension, but even so, are not beyond our attainment if we choose to attain them, and believe that we truly can. (pp. 161-162)

If you live long enough, you will move through fear and on into the deep quiet of what is. Walking away from western medicine meant walking into the unknown for both my husband and me. Some claimed that we were crazy and others applauded our decision. Most remained silent, not knowing what to say and wanting to reclaim their denial that death was not coming to their dear friend — and certainly not to them.

My husband survived his cancer. He beat all the odds by living, but the question remains for us, did he? Neither my husband nor I are the same people we were before his cancer. Indeed there was a death and a rebirth for both of us.

For a while people would call us — people we did not know who had somehow found out about us — to ask in detail what he had done to live, to beat death. All of them had been told they would soon be dead from cancer and they were panicked. It was always hard for them to hear that we had not beaten death but rather had learned to live side by side with death, ready to go and truly ready to live more fully. Certainly we would share the details of what medications and alternative resources we had used but these resources were not the cure. We knew this.

We knew the lesson of impermanence. We experienced a depth of surrender to impermanence, to the mystery of life. How could we teach this concept of impermanence to a person whose whole life was based in denial of impermanence? We spoke often about meditation and prayer to each person who called us; we advised each one to listen from inside.

If you live long enough you will experience liberation from permanence. You might experience impermanence in various forms of your daily life. Perhaps a police officer pulls you over for swerving, not because of alcohol but because your hand is unsteady on the wheel. Your driver's license could be taken away and you would be dependent on public transportation or friends and family to get around. Your choice of reactions is wide and varied. You could resist by being angry, or by being passive aggressive and refusing to go with your assigned driver. Or you could accept. You could enjoy nature as you wait for your ride; you might even meet new people who could be some of the greatest teachers of your life and give you more opportunities to say thank you.

If you live long enough, you will have more opportunities to say thank you.

You might need to wear adult diapers that someone half your age will put on you. You might be fed by someone else. And if you cannot speak, you might learn to say thank you with your eyes or those aged hands whose knotted veins you no longer deny. You might experience gratitude for your hands' sensitivity in helping you through your aging.

If you live long enough, you will become humble. I have held hands with my own death through a near-fatal car accident in1980 and almost drowning in an ocean riptide at age eight. My death has not come yet but it will one day; that is certain. I am humbled that I am still here to tell my story, still here on this earth, working, loving, and sharing with others all the gifts of aging.

If you live long enough, you will tell your story of living, aging, and dying. As you age you will enter the great mystery school where you can take great pleasure in just holding someone's hand for an hour, where you may pee if you laugh heartily, where you find it breathtaking to watch a leaf fall from a tree, where you applaud the great blue heron returning to nest in the same gnarled old tree for the third, fourth, or fifth time.

If you live long enough, you will live in the moment. You may not remember people, places, events, books, yesterday, or the words you just said. You may be lost in a state of consciousness that seems miserable to some and enlightened to others. But you will at times experience deep peace at what is in the moment.

If you live long enough, you will experience isolation and community. You will become more curious about what is happening to you and your friends and family emotionally, physically, and spiritually in the aging process. You might satisfy your curiosity through reading and education in a variety of forums: classes on aging, discussions with friends, meditation, prayer and consulting various professionals to confront your issues of aging. You will begin to understand how much alike we are in aging. And when your turn comes to die, you will embark on one of the greatest journeys of your life, helping those who dearly love you to remember and live the gifts you have given them.

If you live long enough, you will experience gratitude to the authors of this book. Reading a book is a short part of your life's journey and here we are at the end of this short journey together. Endings create space for beginnings. So now is the time to live what matters to you from this book.

If you live long enough, you will awaken to aging and live consciously.

References

Stein, G. (2008). *The art of racing in the rain.* New York: HarperCollins.

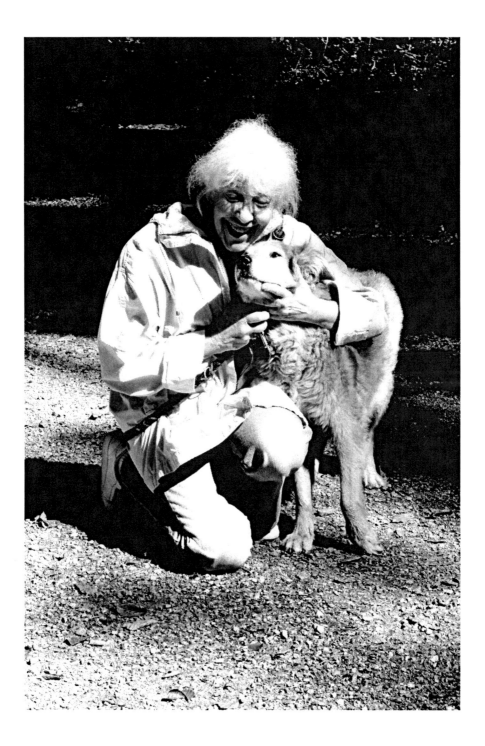

Bibliography

Aging, Death, Dying, Grief Issues

Ajjan, D. (Ed.). (1994). *The day my father dies: Women share their stories of love, loss and life.* Philadelphia: Running Press.

Arrien, A. (2005). *The second half of life: Opening the eight gates of wisdom.* Louisville, CO: Sounds True Press.

Berman, C. (2005). *Caring for yourself while caring for your aging parents.* New York: Henry Holt and Co.

Bolen, J. S. (2003). *Crones don't whine, concentrated wisdom for juicy women.* Newburyport, MA: Conari Press.

Bugental, E. (2005). *Agesong.* San Francisco: Elders Academy Press.

Bugental, E. (2008). *Love fills in the blanks: Paradoxes of our final years.* San Francisco: Elders Academy Press.

Campbell, J. (1986). *The inner reaches of outer space: Metaphor as myth and as religion.* New York: HarperCollins.

Darling, D. (1995). *Soul search: A scientist explores the afterlife.* New York: Villard.

Dass, R., Matousek, M., & Roeder, M. (2001). *Still here: Embracing aging, changing and dying.* Riverhead, NY: Riverhead Press.

de Ropp, R.S. (1968). *The master game.* New York: Dell Publishing.

Erikson, E. H., Erikson, J. M., & Kivnick, H. Q. (1986). *Vital involvement in old age.* New York: Norton.

Foster, R. J. (1992). *Prayer: Finding the heart's true home.* New York: HarperCollins.

Grollman, E. A. (1997). *Living when a loved one has died.* Boston: Beacon Press.

Halifax, J. (2008) *Being with dying, cultivating compassion and fearlessness.* Boston: Shambala.

Jackson, E. (1971). *When someone dies.* Minneapolis, MN: Fortress Press.

James, J. W. & Friedman, R. (1998). *The grief recovery handbook* (Rev. ed.). New York: HarperCollins.

Johnson, E. A. (1995). *As someone dies: Handbook for the living.* Carlsbad, CA: Hay House.

Keleman, S. (1975). *Living your dying.* New York: Random House.

Kreis, B., & Pattie, A. (1982). *Up from grief: Patterns of recovery.* San Francisco: HarperSanFrancisco.

Kubler-Ross, E. (1986). *Death – The final stage of growth.* New York: Touchstone.

Kubler-Ross, E. (1991) *On life after death.* Berkeley: Celestial Arts.

Kubler-Ross, E. (1997*). On death and dying.* New York: Scribner.

Kubler-Ross, E. (1997). *Questions and answers on death and dying.* New York: Scribner.

Kubler-Ross, E. (1997). *To live until we say goodbye.* New York: Scribner.

Levine, S. (1989). *Meetings at the edge: Dialogues with the grieving and dying, healing and healed.* New York: Anchor Books.

Levine, S. (2000). *Who dies?: An investigation of conscious living and conscious dying.* Minneapolis, MN: Gill and Macmillan.

Lipschitz, D. (2002). *Breaking the rules of aging.* Washington, DC: LifeLine Press.

Loverde, J. (2000). *The complete eldercare planner, where to start, which questions to ask and how to find help* (2nd ed.). New York: Three Rivers Press.

McWilliams, Bloomfield, H. H., & Colgrove, M. (1993). *How to survive the loss of a love.* Nashville: Prelude Press.

Moody, R., Jr. (2001). *Life after life.* San Francisco: HarperSanFrancisco.

Nuland, S. B. (1995). *How we die.* New York: Vintage Books.

O'Connor, N. (1994). *Letting go with love.* Tucson, AZ: La Mariposa Press.

Putter, A. M. (1997). *The memorial rituals book for healing and hope.* Amityville, NY: Baywood Publishing.

Remen, R. N. (1996). *Kitchen table wisdom: Stories that heal.* New York: Riverhead.

Remen, R. N. (2000). *My grandfather's blessings: Stories of strength, refuge, and belonging.* New York: Riverhead.

Ring, K. (1984). *Heading toward omega: In search of the meaning of the near-death experience.* New York: Morrow.

Silverman, P. (Ed.). (1987). *The elderly as modern pioneers.* Bloomington, IN: Indiana University Press.

Spence, L. (1997). *Legacy: A step by step guide to writing personal history.* Athens, OH: Swallow Press.

Staudacher, C. (1987). *Beyond grief: A guide for recovery from the death of a loved one.* Oakland, CA: New Harbinger Publications.

Szasz, T. S. (1961). *The myth of mental illness.* New York: Hoeber-Harper.

Tatelbaum, J. (1984). *The courage to grieve.* New York: Harper & Row.

Veninga, R. (1996). *A gift of hope: How we survive our tragedies.* New York: Ballantine Books.

Westberg, G. E. (1979). *Good grief.* Minneapolis, MN: Augsberg Fortress.

Yalom, I. D. (2008). *Staring at the sun.* San Francisco: Jossey-Bass.

Yalom, M. & Yalom, R. S. (2008). The American resting place: 400 years of history through our cemeteries and burial grounds. New York: Houghton Mifflen.

Zadra, D. & Lambert, K. (1995). *Because of you: Thoughts to inspire the people who inspire us.* Havertown, PA: Compendium Publishing & Communications.

Psychological and Spiritual Issues

Blackman, S. (Ed.). (1997). *Graceful exits: How great beings die: Death stories of Tibetan, Hindu and Zen Masters.* Weatherhill.

Boorstein, S. (2002). *Pay attention for goodness sake.* New York: Ballantine Books. Books.

Brazier, D. (1998). *The feeling Buddha.* New York: Fromm International.

Campbell, J. (2001). *Thou art that.* Novato, CA: New World Library.

Chodron, P. (1994). *Start where you are: A Guide to compassionate living.* Boston: Shambhala.

Chodron, P. (2000). *When things fall apart.* Boston: Shambhala.

Chodron, P. (2001). *The places that scare you: A guide to fearlessness in difficult times.* Boston: Shambhala.

Dalai Lama. (2002). *Advice on dying (and living a better life).* Atria Books.

Dass, R. (2000). *Still here.* New York: Penguin Putnam.

Gafni, M. (2001). *Soul prints.* New York: Simon & Schuster.

Hafiz (1999). *The gift: Poems by Hafiz the great Sufi master* (D. Ladinsky, trans.). New York: Penguin Group.

Heschel, A. J. & Dresner, S. H. (Eds). (2004). *I asked for wonder: A spiritual anthology of Abraham Joshua Heschel.* New York: Crossroad.

Kabat-Zinn, J. (1990). *Full catastrophe living: Using the wisdom of your body and mind to face stress pain and illness.* New York: Dell.

Kirvan, J. (2001). *Silent hope: Living with the mystery of God.* Notre Dame, IN: Sorin Books.

Kramer, K. (1988). *The sacred art of dying: How world religions understand death.* Mahwah, NJ: Paulist Press.

Kornfield, J. (2001). *Meditation for beginners.* (Audio CD). Sounds True

Kornfield, J.(2001). *After the ecstasy, the laundry : How the heart grows wise on the spiritual path.* New York: Bantam.

Kornfield, J. (1993). *A path with heart: A guide through the perils and promises of spiritual life.* New York: Bantam.

Kushner, H. (2004). *When bad things happen to good people.* New York: Anchor.

Lamott, A. (2005). *Plan B.* New York: Penguin Group.

Levine, O. & Levine, S. (1982). *Who dies?* Anchor Books.

Lewis, C. S. (2001). *A grief observed.* San Francisco: HarperSanFrancisco.

McCarroll, T. (1994). *Childsong, monksong: A spiritual journey.* New York: St. Martin's Press.

Miller, S. (1997). *After death: Mapping the journey.* New York: Simon & Schuster.

Remen, R. N. (2000). *My Grandfather's blessings.* New York: Penguin Putnam.

Sharp, J. (1996). *Living our dying: A way to the sacred in everyday life.* New York: Hyperion Books.

Singh, K. D. (1998) *The grace in dying: How we are transformed spiritually as we die.* New York: HarperCollins.

Sogyal Rinpoche. (1994). *The Tibetan book of living and dying.* San Francisco: HarperSanFrancisco.

Westberg, G. (2004). *Good grief.* Minneapolis, MN: Augsburg Fortress Publishers.

Wiersbe, W. (1984). *Why us?: When bad things happen to God's people.* Grand Rapids, MI: Fleming H. Revell.

Wilber, K. (2001). *Grace and grit: Spirituality and healing in the life and death of Treya Killam Wilber.* Boston: Shambhala.

Yancey, P. (2001). *Where is God when it hurts?* Grand Rapids, MI: Zondervan.

Tournier, P. (1972). *Learning to grow old.* London: SCM Press Ltd.

Ueshiba, M. (2002). *The art of peace.* (J. Stevens, trans.). Boston: Shambhala Press.

Practical Issues

Esperti, R. & Peterson, R. (1988). *Loving trust: The right way to provide for yourself and guarantee the future of your loved ones.* New York: Viking.

Collier, C. (2002). *Wealth in families.* Cambridge, MA: Harvard Press.

Domini, A. with Pearne, D. & Rich, S. (1988). *Challenges of Wealth.* Dow Jones-Irwin.

Hospice of Petaluma. (n.d.). *Helping people prepare.* Petaluma, CA: Hospice of Petaluma/Memorial Hospice.

Hospice of Petaluma (n.d.). *What to Consider When Planning in Advance.* Petaluma, CA: Hospice of Petaluma/Memorial Hospice

Hospice of Petaluma (n.d.). *When Someone Dies – Resources and Support Services.* Petaluma, CA: Hospice of Petaluma/Memorial Hospice.

Hughes, J. E. Jr. (2004). *Family wealth.* New York: Bloomberg Press.

Levy, J. (2008). *Coping with inherited wealth: Opportunities and dilemmas*. North Charleston, SC: Booksurge Publishing.

Neeleman, S., Garrity, C., & Baris, M. (2003). *Estate planning for the healthy wealthy family.* New York: Allworth Press.

Web Sites

General

www.aarp.org
www.aoa.org Administration on Aging
www.census.gov
cms.hhs.gov/researchers/
www.agingstats.gov/chartbook2000/
www.civicventures.org
www.generationsjournal.org (Narratives on Older Adults)
www.independentsector.org
www.ilcusa.org

Housing Options

www.secondjourney.org/2005Councils.htm
www.edenalt.com/welcome.htm
www.alternativesforseniors.com/descriptAlter.php
www.matherlifeways.com/
www.seniorhousingnet.com/seniors/?source=a2gg7tjt517&refcd=GO0
 SRH00B_senior_housing
thegreenhouseproject.com/concept.html
www.cohousing.org/
www.homemods.org/library/
library.louisville.edu/government/federal/agencies/hud/urbanresear
 ch.html
www.findahousemate.com or email: lfanucchi@HIPhousing.org/
www.peoples-law.org/housing/assisted-housing/homesharing.htm
www.aoa.gov/naic/elderloc.html

Elder Care Options

www.elderweb.com/?PageID=2971
www.eldercarelink.com/
www.elderlivingsource.com/
www.nih.gov/news/NIH-Record/07_29_97/story02.htm
www.ec-online.net/Knowledge/Articles/movingin.html
hr.ucsb.edu/Worklife/Elder_Care/elder_care_familyhomes.htm
www.helpguide.org/elder/senior_housing_residential_care_types.htm
www.usaaedfoundation.org/family/ec03.asp
www.globalaging.org/elderrights/us/2004/teamup.htm
www.globalaging.org/whatsnew/listserv.htm
www.aoa.gov/index.asp

Resolving Elder Issues

www.achievingresolution.com/pg8.cfm
www.commonweal.org
www.hms.harvard.edu/hr/owf_eldercare.html
www.merck.com/mrkshared/mmg/sec1/ch15/ch15g.jsp
worklifebalance.ucdavis.edu/balancing/ea_options.html
www.canhr.org/abuse/abuse_index.html
www.apa.org/pi/aging/eldabuse.html
www.aging-parents-and-elder-
care.com/Pages/Assisted_Living_and_Other.html
www.4woman.gov/violence/elder.cfm
www.asaging.org/index.cfm
/ist-socrates.berkeley.edu/~aging/ResourcesinAging.html
(email ddriver@berkeley.edu to get on mailing list)
www.ucpress.edu/books/pages/8992/8992.ch01.html
www.ppic.org/main/publication.asp?i=309
www.pacificinstitute.org/ev_nord.html
www.jcagency.org/friendship-circle.shtml
www.ncoa.org/content.cfm?sectionID=110&detail=16

Advance Health Care Directives and Dying

www.helpguide.org/elder/advance_directive_end_of_life_care.htm
www.aarp.org/families/end_life
www.nhpco.org
www.funeria.com Ashes to art, urns

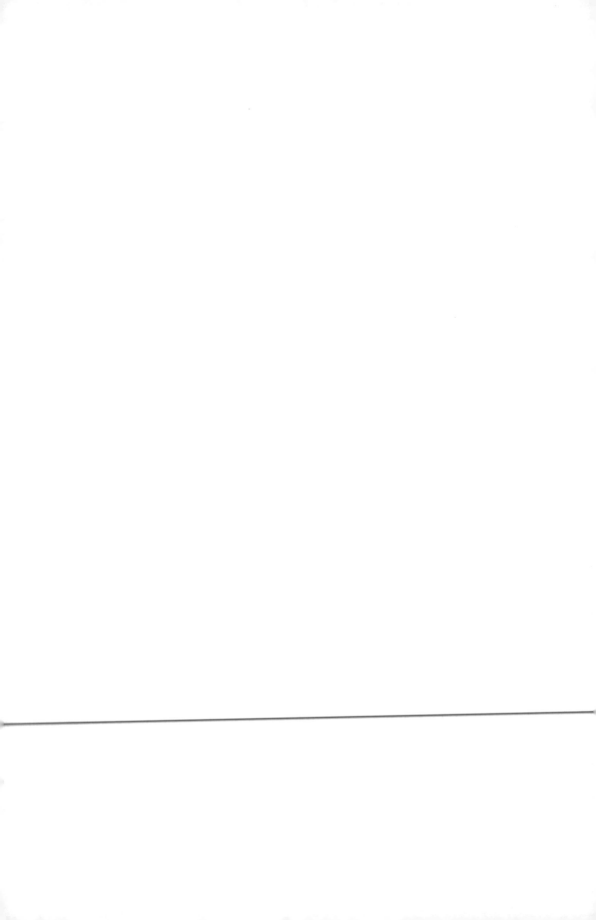

About the Contributors

Elizabeth Bugental, PhD, spent her 20s and 30s as a Roman Catholic nun. She has taught on all levels and was for over a decade the chairperson of the Department of Theatre Arts at Immaculate Heart College in Los Angeles. Her second career, lasting into her sixties, was as a psychotherapist in the San Francisco Bay Area, in private practice and jointly with her husband, James F.T. Bugental, noted psychologist and author. She holds a doctorate from Stanford University in speech and drama, an MA from Catholic University of America, and is a licensed Marriage and Family Therapist in California. She is the author of *AgeSong: Meditations for our Later Years.* For the last six years Elizabeth has been the full-time caretaker for her husband, who suffered from dementia and partial paralysis as the result of a stroke. Jim died peacefully at home with Elizabeth and family, September 18, 2008. She was on the advisory board for the International Institute for Humanistic Studies until her death in February, 2009.

Carol Cook, MA, is a Licensed Professional Therapist. She has had a private practice in Prescott, Arizona for 15 years. Before becoming a therapist she had careers in state government, education and the corporate world. Carol is also a mother, grandmother and great-grandmother. She has had a formal meditation practice since 1992, and has managed Vipassana meditation retreats since 1999. Carol reads and writes poetry to evoke deeper resonance with her daily experiences.

Doug Cort, PhD, is a clinical psychologist and an Associate Clinical Professor in the Department of Internal Medicine at the University of California, Davis. He has directed the Psychology Section of the Preventive Cardiology Program at University of California Davis Medical Center since 1992. He is also the director of psychology services at St. Helena Hospital's Center for Behavioral Health, where he oversees a training program for doctoral students in clinical psychology. Additionally, he maintains a private psychotherapy practice in Vallejo, California. Dr. Cort has lectured widely in the United States and abroad on topics related to health psychology.

Pamela Cronin, MA, licensed marriage and family therapist, is in private practice in Burlingame, CA, where she works with children, families and individuals. After writing her Master's thesis on "Life Satisfaction and the Aging Population" in 1996, she developed a special interest in the aging process and now assists families and individuals who are coping with aging, grief, loss, death and dying. She continues to perform research, to write, and to develop ways for families to nurture mutually beneficial relationships, in the moment, with an awareness of the aging process. Pamela has volunteered at Kara, a non profit organization supporting grief and loss programs for individuals and families who have experienced the death of a loved one. She facilitated uncomplicated and complicated grief and loss support groups which involve death from natural causes, homicide and suicide. She has also volunteered at the Friendship Line, a telephone support system in San Francisco for isolated elders with emotional and medical conditions, and served as volunteer coordinator and community educator at the Center for Domestic Violence Prevention in the mid 1990's. Pamela is on the advisory board of the International Institute for Humanistic Studies.

Rev. Karuna Gerstein was the director of senior services at Petaluma People Services Center bringing a great deal of energy and creativity to the many programs she managed. She also served as a chaplain for Hospice of Napa. In this capacity she accompanied elder and non-elder individuals, couples, families and groups on their spiritual journeys as they faced the end of life. Rev. Gerstein holds a B.A. in interpersonal communication from California State University, Hayward, and is an ordained Interfaith Minister through the Chaplaincy Institute of the Arts and Interfaith Ministries in Berkeley. She currently serves the community as a minister, Spiritual Director/Counselor, Dreamworker and teacher of many spiritual practices. Rev. Gerstein is continually inspired by her relationships with elders and has a particular interest in and commitment to the issues we all face as we age and approach the end of our lives. Her passions manifest in the many ways she advocates for elders, the invisible and under-appreciated populations whom she truly believes have much to teach the rest of us. She is dedicated to fostering that which connects us, while embracing and understanding that which divides us.

Christopher S. M. Grimes, PsyD, worked part-time for Behavioral Health Partners (BHP) in Kansas City, Missouri for the past two years. BHP provides psychological assessment and treatment for elderly individuals living in residential care and nursing home facilities. The staff of psychologists and social workers is lead by President and

Owner, John T. Bopp, Ph.D., and Vice President Margaret Barger, M.A. With a staff of 20 clinicians serving facilities throughout the greater Kansas City area, BHP is a great asset to the Kansas City community. Dr. Grimes worked for BHP two days a week, while maintaining a medium sized case load in an independent group private practice setting three days a week. Recently, Dr. Grimes accepted a position with the Saint Louis Behavioral Medicine Institute where he is now serving as Director of the Program for Psychology and Religion. Dr. Grimes earned a Doctor of Psychology (PsyD) from the Forest Institute of Professional Psychology in 2004.

Sandra Harner, PhD, a clinical psychologist, was a post-doctoral fellow in the psychology section of the Preventive Cardiology Program at University of California Davis Medical Center. Currently, she is the director of health research at the Foundation for Shamanic Studies in Mill Valley. She maintains a private psychotherapy practice specializing in Existential-Humanistic psychotherapy and health psychology in Mill Valley, California. She is on the Advisory Board of International Institute for Humanistic Studies.

Myrtle Heery, PhD, licensed MFT, Associate Professor of Psychology, Sonoma State University, Rohnert Park, CA, Associate Core Faculty, Institute of Transpersonal Psychology, Palo Alto, CA, and Director of the International Institute of Humanistic Studies. She teaches two-year trainings nationally and internationally, titled Unearthing the Moment, which are focused on teaching professionals, and lead to certification of in-depth communication skills in both individual and group settings. She also offers day-long introductory trainings across the U.S. and maintains a private practice in Petaluma, CA, leading consultation groups for therapists and providing therapy to individuals, couples, and families with emphasis on aging issues. She is a volunteer for Hospice of Petaluma for two decades providing bereavement counseling to individuals and groups. She has published papers and chapters in psychology journals and books on bereavement, existential-humanistic and transpersonal psychotherapy and psychology. Over eighteen years ago she accompanied her husband in surviving a cancer protocol giving him three months to live.

Fran Korb, MD, graduated from Wellesley College in 1945 and Cornell Medical School in 1949. She interned at Bellevue Hospital in New York City in pediatrics, and worked for the San Francisco Department of Health with infants and school-age children. She later retired from medical practice, studied family therapy, and practiced as a family therapist until retiring in the early 80's. During her retirement she has volunteered as an environmental teacher for children, grown flowers for commercial drying, worked as a ranger at Point Reyes National Seashore, taught science in elementary schools, and volunteered as a bereavement group leader for Hospice of Petaluma . She moved to Friends House, a retirement community, in 2002.

John L. Levy, MBA, After graduating from Stanford with a BA in Engineering and an MBA, punctuated by service in the U.S. Navy during World War 2, he spent ten years in heavy construction with Bechtel Corporation. He received an inheritance which enabled him to spend the rest of his professional career in non-profit organizations devoted to psychological and spiritual issues, first as a volunteer and later, when his inheritance was nearly spent, in paid positions. Organizations he worked in include Sequoia Seminar, the American Friends Service Committee, San Francisco Venture, the Association for Humanistic Psychology (as Executive Officer), the C.G. Jung Institute of San Francisco (as Executive Director) and the California Institute of Integral Studies (as Interim Provost). For the past 25 years he has had a private practice working with individuals and families on issues involving inherited wealth. He made presentations and led discussions for financial planners, estate planning attorneys, family office managers, bank trust officers, investment advisors, psychotherapists and other professionals. He recently published a book, "Inherited Wealth: Opportunities and Dilemmas" based on articles he has written over the years.

Laura Michaels is an Environmental Studies and Planning graduate of Sonoma State University (SSU) and has recently completed an SSU Certificate Program in Gerontology. From 2004-2006, Laura served on the Senior Safety Fall Prevention Task Force for the County of Sonoma, CA., where she organized and led countywide "Safe Steps" workshops for seniors. Laura has worked as a case manager at Sonoma Kinship Family Center, where she provided services and resources for grandparents and other kinship caregivers who are raising their relative's children. She was a member of the Caregiver's Support Group led by Elizabeth and Jim Bugental.

Bev Miller, Grief Services Educator, has been associated with Hospice of Petaluma since 1984, three years after the death of her husband. At the time of his death she prayed that God would not only get her through all that was facing her—single parenting, running a business, surviving financial crisis—but also help her understand what in the world this parenthesis in her life meant. She studied what scripture had to say about "waiting on God" and thus began a three-year path toward hospice ministry. She began as a volunteer shortly before the decision was made by Hospice of Petaluma to expand its Grief Support Services, and served as a volunteer in care giving and grief support until 1987, when she was offered a position as Assistant Bereavement Services coordinator. She has been involved with Hospice of Petaluma on some level ever since, as a volunteer and staff member primarily in bereavement, but also at times with caregiving, administration, fund raising and the capital campaign for building the new facility. Her primary role now is the management and supervision of adult grief support groups. She is on the board of the International Institute for Humanistic Studies.

Regina Reilly, MS, licensed MFT, is a teacher of the Diamond Approach, a method of inquiry and a path of spiritual transformation originated by A.H. Almaas. She lives and works in the San Francisco bay area of California and has been in private practice of psychotherapy for three decades. From 1981 to 1986, she was the co-founder and director of the Transpersonal Counseling Center in Oakland, California where she trained students of John F. Kennedy University to become therapists with a spiritual perspective. She is a writer and a member of the advisory board of the International Institute of Humanistic Studies.

Gregg Richardson, PhD, licensed clinical psychologist, holds MAs in comparative literature and religious studies from Indiana University, Bloomington, and an MA and PhD in clinical psychology from the California Institute of Integral Studies (CIIS, San Francisco, with post-doctoral training in gerontology and adult neuropsychology. He has taught at CIIS, the Saybrook Institute (San Francisco), and the Wright Institute (Berkeley), as well as in Russia and Taiwan. He spent ten years in AIDS support work in San Francisco in the 1990s, and four years as graduate advisor for the doctoral psychology program at CIIS. He has practiced clinical neuropsychology at two Kaiser hospitals in the San Francisco Bay Area over the past ten years, specializing in adult neurocognitive assessment and adult attention deficit disorder. He has also served as president of AHIMSA, a Bay-Area organization promoting non-violence, and authored articles on AIDS, non-violence, aging and menopause. Gregg is on the advisory board of the International Institute for Humanistic Studies.

Will Rogers, Attorney at Law, graduated from the University of California, Berkeley, in 1988 with a degree in rhetoric, and from the University of California Hastings College of Law in 1991. Since then, he has maintained a law practice in the San Francisco Bay Area. He has also been deeply engaged in spiritual practice for over 30 years. Part of his current spiritual discipline consists in applying the insights gained from his inner work to the practical problems and needs of his clients. He is on the board of the International Institute for Humanistic Studies. Will and his wife homeschooled their son through all his schooling until his enrollment in college. Will is grateful to his wife for helping him discover the depths of his heart and for reminding him that everything comes from the One.

Barbara Sapienza, PhD, is a clinical psychologist in private practice in San Francisco and Corte Madera. She is affiliated with the San Francisco Psychotherapy Research Clinic and Training program as a teacher and supervisor. She has presented at aging seminar at International Institute for Humanistic Studies, 2007. She works, writes, and paints, nourished by her family and friends. Her grandchildren, Milla and Isabella, are her teachers and guide her path in many ways. This Chapter is an excerpt from a memoir in progress.

Hobart F. "Red" Thomas, PhD, is professor emeritus of psychology at Sonoma State University, and one of the founding members of the psychology department at Sonoma State College in 1961. Nine years later, while teaching at Sonoma State, he became the provost and one of the original founders of the School of Expressive Arts. He has published over fifteen articles in various professional journals, newsletters, bulletins, and reviews, and is also an accomplished jazz pianist. One of the questions he has been exploring is how, in academic settings, to help people get through academic mine fields without losing their humanity. He was a member of the advisory board of the International Institute for Humanistic Studies and Professor Emeritus for the institute until his death, June, 2009.

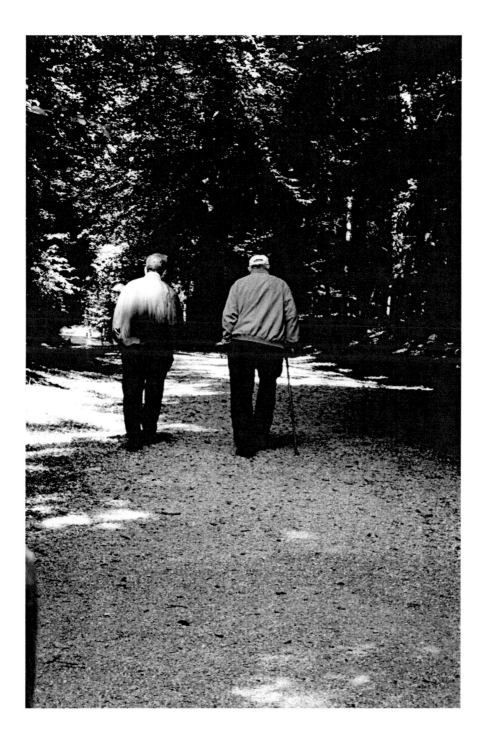

Notes on Aging

Notes on Aging

Notes on Aging

Notes on Aging

Notes on Aging